Introduction to Home Remedies

Home remedies are time-tested, natural, and often simple solutions that have been used for generations to address various health concerns and everyday ailments. These remedies make use of readily available ingredients from our kitchens, gardens, and natural surroundings. While they may not replace professional medical advice or treatment for serious conditions, home remedies can offer relief for minor discomforts and promote a holistic approach to wellness.

The practice of home remedies is deeply rooted in cultural traditions, folk wisdom, and the idea that the body has an innate ability to heal itself. From soothing a sore throat with honey and lemon to using aloe vera to alleviate sunburn, these remedies often draw on the inherent properties of plants, herbs, minerals, and other natural substances.

One of the appealing aspects of home remedies is their accessibility. Many people find comfort in knowing that they can turn to familiar ingredients to create simple yet effective solutions for common ailments. Whether it's using a warm saltwater gargle to ease a scratchy throat or applying aloe vera gel to calm irritated skin, these remedies empower individuals to take an active role in their well-being.

It's important to approach home remedies with a balanced perspective. While they can offer relief and support, they are not a substitute for professional medical care when needed. It's wise to exercise caution, especially if you have allergies, sensitivities, or pre-existing health conditions. Consulting a healthcare professional before trying a new home remedy is advisable, particularly for individuals who are pregnant, nursing, or on medications.

In this age of modern medicine, the wisdom of traditional practices still holds its value. Home remedies bridge the gap between the ancient wisdom of natural healing and our contemporary understanding of health. Whether it's using the healing power of herbal teas, the soothing touch of essential oils, or the nourishment of nutrient-rich foods, home remedies offer a glimpse into the time-honored ways our ancestors cared for themselves and their families.

Home remedies are natural treatments or solutions that people use to address various health issues or minor ailments. These remedies often make use of easily available ingredients from the kitchen or garden. Keep in mind that while home remedies can offer relief for certain minor issues, they are not a substitute for professional medical advice and treatment. If you have a serious medical condition, it's always best to consult a healthcare professional.

Home remedies encompass a wide range of natural treatments and solutions that can be used to address various health issues and everyday concerns. Here are some common types of home remedies:

Herbal Remedies: Utilizing the therapeutic properties of herbs and plants to treat ailments and promote wellness. This can include herbal teas, tinctures, poultices, and more.

Kitchen Ingredients: Making use of everyday items found in the kitchen for various health purposes. Examples include honey, lemon, ginger, garlic, and turmeric.

Topical Treatments: Applying natural substances directly to the skin to alleviate conditions such as burns, rashes, insect bites, and minor wounds.

Inhalation Therapy: Inhaling steam infused with essential oils or herbs to relieve congestion, respiratory issues, and sinus discomfort.

Dietary Changes: Adjusting your diet to include specific foods that are known for their health benefits, such as incorporating more fruits, vegetables, and whole grains.

Hydrotherapy: Using water in different temperatures and forms (cold compresses, warm baths) for therapeutic purposes, like reducing muscle pain or promoting relaxation.

Lifestyle Modifications: Implementing changes in daily habits to improve health, such as practicing meditation for stress reduction or maintaining a regular sleep schedule.

Natural Substances: Using natural substances like salt, baking soda, and vinegar for cleaning, exfoliation, and various household purposes.

Aromatherapy: Using essential oils or aromatic compounds to improve psychological and physical well-being through inhalation or massage.

Physical Manipulation: Utilizing techniques like acupressure, reflexology, and stretching to alleviate pain, stimulate circulation, and promote relaxation.

Homeopathic Remedies: Following the principles of homeopathy, which involves using highly diluted substances to stimulate the body's natural healing processes.

Mind-Body Practices: Engaging in activities like yoga, meditation, and deep breathing exercises to promote mental and emotional well-being.

DIY Beauty and Skincare: Creating homemade masks, scrubs, and treatments using natural ingredients for healthier skin and hair.

Teeth and Mouth Care: Using natural solutions like oil pulling, saltwater rinses, and herbal mouthwashes for oral hygiene and gum health.

Naturopathic Remedies: Following principles of naturopathy, which emphasizes the body's ability to heal itself using natural therapies, lifestyle adjustments, and holistic approaches.

Folk Remedies: Traditional practices passed down through generations that often incorporate cultural knowledge and local resources.

It's important to note that while home remedies can provide relief for minor ailments and support well-being, serious or chronic health issues should be addressed with professional medical guidance. Always use caution and consider consulting a healthcare professional before trying any new home remedy, especially if you have allergies, sensitivities, or underlying health conditions.

Herbal remedies

Herbal remedies, also known as herbal medicine or phytotherapy, refer to the use of plants and plant-derived substances for therapeutic purposes to promote health, alleviate symptoms, and prevent or treat various ailments. These remedies have been practiced for centuries across cultures and civilizations as a natural approach to healing and wellness. Herbal remedies make use of the medicinal properties found in different parts of plants, including leaves, flowers, roots, bark, and seeds.

Here's a detailed overview of herbal remedies:

Historical Context:

Herbal remedies have a rich history that spans across ancient civilizations like Traditional Chinese Medicine, Ayurveda, Greek medicine, Indigenous healing traditions, and more. These practices were founded on the belief that nature provides a bounty of remedies for human well-being.

Therapeutic Principles:

Herbal remedies are based on the belief that plants contain bioactive compounds with specific properties that can influence the body's systems and functions. These compounds can include alkaloids, flavonoids, terpenes, essential oils, and more.

Preparation Methods:

Herbal remedies are prepared using different methods to extract or harness the beneficial compounds from plants:

Infusions: Making teas by steeping plant parts in hot water.

Decoctions: Boiling plant parts to extract compounds.

Tinctures: Extracting plant constituents using alcohol or other solvents.

Salves and Ointments: Mixing herbs with carrier oils or beeswax for topical application.

Essential Oils: Distilling plant materials to capture their volatile oils.

Poultices and Compresses: Applying crushed or mashed herbs directly to the skin.

Capsules and Tablets: Drying and encapsulating herbs for convenient consumption.

Common Uses: Herbal remedies can address a wide range of health concerns, including but not limited to:

Digestive issues (e.g., indigestion, bloating)

Respiratory problems (e.g., cough, congestion)

Sleep disturbances and stress

Skin conditions (e.g., acne, eczema)

Pain management

Immune system support

Hormonal balance

Cardiovascular health

Cognitive function and memory

Menstrual and reproductive health

Benefits and Considerations: Holistic Approach: Herbal remedies often consider the whole person and focus on addressing the underlying causes of symptoms.

Gentle and Nurturing: Many herbal remedies are considered milder and gentler than pharmaceutical interventions, making them suitable for minor ailments and sensitive individuals.

Cultural Significance: Herbal practices are deeply rooted in cultural traditions and have been passed down through generations.

Individual Variability: Responses to herbal remedies can vary, and what works for one person might not work for another.

Safety: While generally safe, herbal remedies can interact with medications or cause adverse reactions, making professional guidance crucial.

Research and Evidence: The scientific research on herbal remedies varies. Some herbs have been extensively studied, while others have limited scientific validation.

The effectiveness of herbal remedies can be influenced by factors like the specific plant used, the preparation method, dosage, and individual differences.

Professional Guidance: Consulting a qualified healthcare professional or herbalist is recommended before starting any herbal regimen, especially if you have underlying health conditions, are pregnant, nursing, or taking medications.

Herbal remedies offer a natural and holistic approach to health and well-being. They draw upon the wisdom of traditional practices and the abundant healing properties found in nature's pharmacy. While they can provide support for minor ailments and promote overall wellness, it's important to approach herbal remedies with respect, caution, and the guidance of qualified experts.

100 herbal remedy tips for various health and well-being concerns. Remember to use these tips with caution, and consult a healthcare professional if you have any underlying medical conditions or concerns.

Certainly, here are 50 herbal remedy tips for various health and well-being concerns. Remember to use these tips with caution, and consult a healthcare professional if you have any underlying medical conditions or concerns.

1. **Chamomile Tea for Relaxation:** Sip on chamomile tea before bed to promote relaxation and improve sleep quality.
2. **Peppermint Oil for Headaches**: Dilute peppermint oil and apply it to your temples for relief from tension headaches.
3. **Ginger for Nausea**: Consume ginger tea or ginger candies to alleviate nausea and motion sickness.
4. **Lavender Essential Oil for Stress:** Diffuse lavender oil or add a few drops to your bath for stress relief and relaxation.
5. **Eucalyptus Steam for Congestion**: Inhale eucalyptus steam to clear nasal congestion and ease breathing.
6. **Calendula Salve for Skin Irritations**: Apply calendula salve to soothe minor skin irritations and cuts.
7. **Echinacea Tea for Immune Support:** Drink echinacea tea to boost your immune system during cold and flu season.
8. **Lemon Balm for Anxiety:** Brew lemon balm tea to calm nerves and reduce anxiety.
9. **Turmeric for Inflammation**: Add turmeric to your meals for its anti-inflammatory benefits.
10. **Aloe Vera Gel for Sunburn**: Apply aloe vera gel to sunburned skin for cooling relief and healing.

11. **Nettle Tea for Allergies**: Drink nettle tea to alleviate seasonal allergies and hay fever symptoms.
12. **Cayenne Pepper for Pain:** Create a cayenne pepper salve to reduce muscle and joint pain.
13. **Valerian Root for Sleep:** Take valerian root in supplement form to improve sleep quality.
14. **Fennel Seeds for Digestion:** Chew on fennel seeds after meals to aid digestion and reduce bloating.
15. **Thyme Infusion for Sore Throat:** Gargle with thyme-infused water to soothe a sore throat.
16. **Oregano Oil for Immunity**: Take oregano oil capsules for immune system support.
17. **Hibiscus Tea for Blood Pressure**: Drink hibiscus tea to help lower blood pressure.
18. **Dandelion Root Tea for Detox:** Sip dandelion root tea to support liver detoxification.
19. **Rosemary Oil for Hair Growth**: Mix rosemary essential oil with a carrier oil and massage into your scalp to promote hair growth.
20. **Garlic for Cold Prevention:** Consume raw garlic or add it to dishes to help prevent colds.
21. **Licorice Root for Digestive Health**: Drink licorice root tea to soothe digestive discomfort and support gut health.
22. **Green Tea for Antioxidants:** Enjoy green tea for its rich antioxidants and potential health benefits.
23. **Sage Gargle for Mouth Infections**: Gargle with sage-infused water to treat mouth infections and sore throats.
24. **Olive Leaf Extract for Immunity:** Take olive leaf extract for immune system support.
25. **Fenugreek Seeds for Blood Sugar:** Consume fenugreek seeds to help regulate blood sugar levels.
26. **Marshmallow Root Tea for Coughs:** Drink marshmallow root tea to soothe coughs and throat irritation.
27. **Yarrow for Wound Healing:** Apply crushed yarrow leaves to wounds to promote healing.
28. **Cinnamon for Blood Sugar:** Sprinkle cinnamon on your meals to help stabilize blood sugar.

29. **Ginseng for Energy:** Take ginseng supplements to boost energy and combat fatigue.
30. **Mullein Leaf for Respiratory Health:** Use mullein leaf tea to ease respiratory congestion and promote lung health.
31. **Black Cohosh for Menopause:** Take black cohosh to alleviate menopausal symptoms.
32. **Plantain Leaf for Bug Bites**: Apply crushed plantain leaves to bug bites for itching relief.
33. **Goldenrod Tea for UTIs:** Drink goldenrod tea to support urinary tract health.
34. **Milk Thistle for Liver Support**: Take milk thistle supplements for liver detoxification.
35. **St. John's Wort for Mood**: Use St. John's Wort to manage mild mood imbalances.
36. **Saw Palmetto for Prostate Health**: Take saw palmetto supplements for prostate health in men.
37. **Hawthorn Berry for Heart Health**: Consume hawthorn berry supplements for cardiovascular support.
38. **Echinacea and Goldenseal Combo**: Combine echinacea and goldenseal for immune system enhancement.
39. **Ginger and Honey for Cold Relief**: Mix ginger and honey in warm water to alleviate cold symptoms.
40. **Lemon Balm for Cold Sores**: Apply lemon balm ointment to cold sores for healing.
41. **Nettle Leaf for Hair Health:** Use nettle leaf rinse as a natural hair conditioner for shine and strength.
42. **Red Clover Tea for Skin**: Drink red clover tea for its potential skin-clearing properties.
43. **Catnip for Insomnia:** Brew catnip tea to promote relaxation and aid sleep.
44. **Passionflower for Anxiety:** Consume passionflower tea or supplements for anxiety relief.
45. **Juniper Berry for Urinary Health**: Take juniper berry supplements to support urinary health.
46. **Ginger and Lemon for Digestive Aid:** Combine ginger and lemon juice in warm water as a digestive tonic.
47. **Peppermint for IBS:** Use peppermint oil capsules to alleviate symptoms of irritable bowel syndrome (IBS).

48. **Chamomile and Lavender Bath**: Add chamomile and lavender essential oils to a warm bath for relaxation.
49. **Feverfew for Migraines:** Take feverfew supplements to reduce the frequency and severity of migraines.
50. **Arnica Salve for Bruises:** Apply arnica salve to bruises and sore muscles for healing.
51. **Comfrey Poultice for Sprains:** Create a poultice using comfrey leaves to alleviate pain and inflammation from sprains.
52. **Lemon Verbena Tea for Digestion**: Brew lemon verbena tea to aid digestion and relieve indigestion.
53. **Burdock Root Detox Tea:** Drink burdock root tea to support detoxification and cleanse the body.
54. **Cilantro for Heavy Metal Detox:** Consume cilantro to assist in removing heavy metals from the body.
55. **Yarrow Infusion for Menstrual Cramps:** Drink yarrow infusion to ease menstrual cramps and regulate periods.
56. **Cleavers Tea for Lymphatic Health**: Consume cleavers tea to promote lymphatic drainage and overall detoxification.
57. **Rosehip Oil for Skin Regeneration**: Apply rosehip oil to scars and wrinkles for skin regeneration.
58. **Kava Kava for Relaxation:** Take kava kava supplements for anxiety reduction and relaxation.
59. **Lemongrass for Fever**: Brew lemongrass tea to help reduce fever and induce sweating.
60. **Basil Essential Oil for Focus:** Diffuse basil essential oil to improve concentration and mental clarity.
61. **Valerian and Lemon Balm Combo for Sleep:** Combine valerian and lemon balm for enhanced sleep support.
62. **Bergamot Essential Oil for Mood:** Inhale bergamot oil to uplift mood and reduce stress.
63. **Chickweed Salve for Skin Itching:** Apply chickweed salve to soothe itching and irritation.
64. **Mugwort for Dream Enhancement:** Drink mugwort tea before bed for potentially vivid dreams.
65. **Yellow Dock Root for Iron Absorption:** Consume yellow dock root to support iron absorption in the body.

66. **Hyssop Tea for Respiratory Health:** Brew hyssop tea to help alleviate respiratory congestion and cough.
67. **Angelica Root for Digestive Issues:** Use angelica root to aid digestion and reduce bloating.
68. **Raspberry Leaf Tea for Pregnancy:** Drink raspberry leaf tea during pregnancy to strengthen the uterus and ease labor.
69. **Senna Leaf Tea for Constipation:** Consume senna leaf tea to relieve occasional constipation.
70. **Maca Root for Hormone Balance:** Take maca root supplements to support hormonal balance.
71. **Licorice Root for Adrenal Support:** Use licorice root to promote adrenal gland health and energy balance.
72. **Cat's Claw for Joint Health:** Take cat's claw supplements to support joint mobility and reduce inflammation.
73. **Bupleurum Root for Liver Cleansing**: Consume bupleurum root to aid in liver detoxification.
74. **Juniper Berry Oil for Skin Health:** Apply diluted juniper berry oil to acne-prone skin for its antimicrobial properties.
75. **Hops for Restlessness:** Brew hops tea to alleviate restlessness and promote relaxation.
76. **Saw Palmetto for Hair Loss**: Use saw palmetto supplements to address hair loss in men and women.
77. **Yellowroot Mouthwash for Oral Health:** Prepare yellowroot mouthwash for gum health and oral hygiene.
78. **Angelica Root Oil for Muscle Pain:** Massage angelica root oil onto sore muscles for relief.
79. **Horehound Cough Drops:** Prepare homemade horehound cough drops to ease coughing.
80. **Gymnema Sylvestre for Sugar Cravings:** Take gymnema sylvestre supplements to reduce sugar cravings.
81. **Lomatium Root for Immune Health:** Use lomatium root supplements to support immune function.
82. **Dong Quai for Menstrual Health:** Take dong quai supplements for menstrual cycle balance.
83. **Gota Kola for Cognitive Function:** Consume gota kola to enhance cognitive function and memory.

84. **Reishi Mushroom for Stress:** Take reishi mushroom supplements to manage stress and support relaxation.
85. **Sage Tea for Excessive Sweating**: Drink sage tea to help control excessive sweating.
86. **Ginger and Honey for Cough:** Mix ginger and honey in warm water to soothe coughs.
87. **Horsetail for Hair and Nail Health**: Consume horsetail tea for healthier hair and nails.
88. **White Willow Bark for Pain**: Brew white willow bark tea for natural pain relief.
89. **Chickweed Tea for Weight Management:** Drink chickweed tea to support weight management.
90. **Burdock Root for Skin Conditions**: Consume burdock root to address skin conditions like acne and eczema.
91. **Sarsaparilla for Skin Health:** Take sarsaparilla supplements for clearer skin.
92. **Squawvine for Female Reproductive Health:** Use squawvine supplements for female reproductive support.
93. **White Pine Bark for Respiratory Health**: Brew white pine bark tea to soothe respiratory issues.
94. **Linden Flower Tea for Relaxation:** Drink linden flower tea to promote relaxation and calmness.
95. **Devil's Claw for Joint Discomfort:** Take devil's claw supplements to ease joint discomfort.
96. **Korean Ginseng for Stamina:** Consume Korean ginseng to enhance physical stamina and endurance.
97. **Pau d'Arco for Immune Support:** Use pau d'arco tea or supplements to boost immune function.
98. **Red Clover for Menopause Symptoms:** Drink red clover tea to alleviate menopausal symptoms.
99. **Mint Tea for Digestive Comfort:** Brew mint tea to ease indigestion and gastrointestinal discomfort.
100. **Mullein Oil for Ear Infections:** Use mullein-infused oil drops for earache relief and ear infections.

As with any herbal remedies, it's important to use caution and consult a healthcare professional before incorporating new herbs or supplements into your routine, especially if you have underlying health conditions or are taking medications. Individual responses to herbs can vary, and professional guidance ensures safe and effective usage.

Kitchen Ingredients

"**Kitchen Ingredients**" as a type of home remedy refers to the everyday items commonly found in your kitchen that can be used to address various health and well-being concerns. These ingredients are readily available, easily accessible, and often have therapeutic properties due to their nutritional content, antioxidants, and other bioactive compounds. Utilizing kitchen ingredients as home remedies is a practical and cost-effective way to promote health and alleviate minor discomforts. Here's a more detailed explanation:

Accessible Solutions: Kitchen ingredients are items you likely have in your pantry, refrigerator, or spice rack. They eliminate the need to make special purchases for home remedies, making them convenient for immediate use.

Nutrient-Rich Benefits: Many kitchen ingredients are rich in vitamins, minerals, and antioxidants that contribute to overall health. For example:

Honey contains enzymes, vitamins, and antioxidants.
Garlic is known for its immune-boosting properties.
Turmeric contains curcumin, a powerful anti-inflammatory compound.
Lemon is a good source of vitamin C and can aid digestion.
Ginger has anti-nausea and anti-inflammatory effects.

Versatile Applications: Kitchen ingredients can be used in various ways, such as:

Ingesting them as part of your diet or as teas.
Applying them topically to the skin.
Combining them with other ingredients to create remedies.

Common Kitchen Remedies:

Honey and Lemon for Sore Throat: Combining honey and lemon in warm water can soothe a sore throat.
Ginger Tea for Nausea: Ginger tea made from fresh ginger root can alleviate nausea.
Oatmeal for Skin Irritation: Applying colloidal oatmeal to the skin can soothe itching and irritation.
Baking Soda for Heartburn: Mixing baking soda in water can help alleviate heartburn.
Apple Cider Vinegar for Digestion: Drinking diluted apple cider vinegar can aid digestion.
Banana for Muscle Cramps: Eating bananas can help prevent muscle cramps due to their potassium content.

Culinary and Health Benefits: Many kitchen ingredients are not only used for health remedies but also add flavor and depth to culinary dishes. This dual use makes incorporating them into your routine more enjoyable.

Cautions and Considerations: While kitchen ingredients are generally safe for most people, it's important to remember:

Allergies: Some individuals may be allergic to specific ingredients.
Dosage: Even natural ingredients can have side effects if consumed in excessive amounts.
Interactions: Certain kitchen ingredients might interact with medications or affect certain health conditions.

Holistic Approach: Using kitchen ingredients as home remedies is part of a holistic approach to wellness. It acknowledges the connection between what you consume and how it impacts your overall health.

Incorporating kitchen ingredients into your home remedy toolkit can empower you to proactively address minor health issues and promote well-being without the need for elaborate preparations or specialized products. However, if you have specific health concerns or are on medication, it's advisable to consult a healthcare professional before relying solely on kitchen ingredients for treatment.

Here are **100 tips** for using kitchen ingredients to support your health and well-being as part of home remedies:

Immune Support:

1. Start your day with a glass of warm water and lemon juice to boost digestion and immunity.
2. Consume garlic regularly for its immune-boosting properties.
3. Make a turmeric and ginger tea to reduce inflammation and support immunity.
4. Include probiotic-rich yogurt in your diet for gut health and immunity.
5. Add honey to herbal teas to soothe a sore throat and provide antioxidants.

Digestive Health:

6. Sip on peppermint tea to alleviate indigestion and bloating.
7. Mix ginger and honey in warm water to ease nausea and aid digestion.
8. Eat fiber-rich foods like oats and fruits to promote healthy digestion.
9. Use fennel seeds as a post-meal digestive aid to prevent gas and discomfort.
10. Consume papaya to support digestion due to its enzyme content.

Skin Care:

11. Create a honey and oatmeal face mask to soothe and moisturize your skin.
12. Apply coconut oil as a natural moisturizer for soft and hydrated skin.
13. Use apple cider vinegar as a toner to balance skin pH and reduce acne.
14. Make a turmeric and yogurt mask to brighten and improve skin complexion.
15. Apply aloe vera gel to sunburned skin for cooling relief and healing.

Hair Health:

16. Massage olive oil into your scalp to nourish and condition your hair.
17. Rinse your hair with diluted apple cider vinegar to restore shine and pH balance.
18. Create a hair mask with mashed avocado to promote hair health and hydration.
19. Apply yogurt to your hair as a natural conditioner to add moisture and shine.
20. Use a mixture of egg yolk and olive oil as a deep conditioning treatment.

Respiratory Health:

21. Inhale steam infused with eucalyptus oil to clear nasal congestion.
22. Drink warm water with honey and lemon to soothe a sore throat and cough.
23. Brew thyme tea to ease respiratory congestion and support lung health.
24. Consume onions and garlic to help relieve congestion during colds.
25. Add turmeric to your diet to support respiratory health and reduce inflammation.

Stress Relief:

26. Sip on chamomile tea to relax and reduce stress and anxiety.
27. Diffuse lavender essential oil to promote relaxation and improve sleep quality.
28. Practice deep breathing exercises using essential oils like bergamot or frankincense.
29. Consume dark chocolate in moderation for its mood-enhancing properties.

Bone Health:

30. Incorporate omega-3-rich foods like walnuts and flaxseeds to support brain health.
31. Include dairy products, leafy greens, and fortified foods for calcium intake.
32. Consume vitamin D-rich foods like fatty fish, egg yolks, and fortified milk.
33. Snack on almonds for their magnesium content, which supports bone health.
34. Incorporate broccoli and Brussels sprouts to enhance your vitamin K intake.
35. Enjoy citrus fruits and bell peppers for their vitamin C contribution to bone health.

Heart Health:

36. Cook with olive oil to benefit from its heart-healthy monounsaturated fats.
37. Eat fatty fish like salmon for omega-3 fatty acids that support heart health.
38. Add garlic to your meals to help lower blood pressure and support circulation.
39. Snack on nuts like walnuts and almonds for their heart-protective benefits.
40. Include oats in your diet to help lower cholesterol levels.

Weight Management:

41. Use smaller plates to help control portion sizes and prevent overeating.
42. Choose high-fiber foods like beans, lentils, and whole grains to promote fullness.
43. Incorporate protein-rich foods like lean meats, beans, and yogurt for satiety.
44. Snack on fruits and vegetables for low-calorie, nutrient-dense options.
45. Stay hydrated by drinking water throughout the day to support metabolism.

Joint and Muscle Health:

46. Add turmeric to your cooking to reduce inflammation and support joint health.
47. Eat foods rich in vitamin C like oranges and strawberries to aid collagen production.
48. Incorporate ginger into your diet to help reduce muscle soreness and inflammation.
49. Consume fatty fish to benefit from omega-3 fatty acids' anti-inflammatory effects.
50. Stay hydrated to support joint lubrication and overall muscle function.

Cognitive Function:

51. Eat a variety of colorful fruits and vegetables for their antioxidants and brain health benefits.
52. Include foods rich in antioxidants like blueberries and spinach to support cognitive function.
53. Consume nuts and seeds for their vitamin E content, which promotes brain health.
54. Incorporate whole grains like quinoa and brown rice for sustained energy and brain function.
55. Enjoy green tea for its caffeine and antioxidants that can enhance alertness.

Blood Sugar Management:

56. Opt for whole grains like oats and quinoa to help stabilize blood sugar levels.

57. Consume cinnamon to improve insulin sensitivity and aid blood sugar control.
58. Include high-fiber foods like legumes and vegetables to slow down glucose absorption.
59. Eat lean protein sources like chicken, fish, and tofu to prevent blood sugar spikes.
60. Choose low-glycemic index fruits like berries and apples for better blood sugar regulation.

Antioxidant Boost:

61. Snack on nuts like almonds and walnuts for their antioxidant content.
62. Enjoy berries like blueberries, strawberries, and raspberries for their high antioxidant levels.
63. Add spinach and kale to your diet for their powerful antioxidant properties.
64. Consume green tea to benefit from its catechins, potent antioxidants.
65. Include colorful vegetables like bell peppers and tomatoes to diversify your antioxidant intake.

Detoxification Support:

66. Drink plenty of water throughout the day to support kidney function and detoxification.
67. Include cruciferous vegetables like broccoli and cauliflower to aid liver detoxification.
68. Consume fiber-rich foods like beans and whole grains to promote regular bowel movements.
69. Add lemon slices to your water to enhance detoxification and hydration.
70. Eat beets to support liver health and enhance detox processes.

Anti-Inflammatory Choices:

71. Cook with olive oil to benefit from its anti-inflammatory monounsaturated fats.
72. Include fatty fish like salmon, mackerel, and sardines for their omega-3 fatty acids.
73. Consume leafy greens like spinach and kale for their anti-inflammatory properties.
74. Add garlic and turmeric to your meals to reduce inflammation.

75. Incorporate nuts and seeds to benefit from their anti-inflammatory nutrients.

Balanced Hormones:

76. Eat foods rich in omega-3 fatty acids to support hormonal balance.
77. Include flaxseeds and chia seeds for their lignans, which can help balance hormones.
78. Consume cruciferous vegetables like broccoli and cauliflower to aid estrogen metabolism.
79. Opt for whole grains to support stable blood sugar levels and hormonal health.
80. Enjoy pumpkin seeds for their zinc content, which supports hormone production.

Energy Boost:

81. Choose complex carbohydrates like whole grains and sweet potatoes for sustained energy.
82. Snack on nuts and seeds for their protein and healthy fats to keep you energized.
83. Consume bananas for a quick source of natural energy from carbohydrates.
84. Incorporate lean protein sources like chicken, fish, and beans to support energy levels.
85. Drink green tea for a mild caffeine boost and antioxidants that promote alertness.

Bone Health:

86. Consume dairy products like milk, yogurt, and cheese for their calcium content.
87. Eat leafy greens like kale and collard greens to boost your vitamin K intake.
88. Enjoy fatty fish like salmon and sardines for their vitamin D and omega-3 fatty acids.
89. Opt for fortified foods like orange juice and cereal to enhance your bone health.
90. Include magnesium-rich foods like nuts, seeds, and whole grains to support bone density.

Hydration:

91. Drink water throughout the day to stay hydrated and support bodily functions.
92. Consume water-rich fruits and vegetables like cucumbers, watermelon, and celery.
93. Brew herbal teas like chamomile or mint for hydration without added calories.
94. Eat soups and broths made from nutrient-rich vegetables for hydration and nourishment.
95. Infuse water with slices of citrus fruits, berries, or herbs for flavor and hydration.

Healthy Snacking:

96. Snack on carrot and celery sticks with hummus for a satisfying and nutrient-rich option.
97. Enjoy Greek yogurt with berries and a drizzle of honey for a balanced snack.
98. Choose whole fruits like apples, pears, and bananas for convenient and wholesome snacking.
99. Create a trail mix with nuts, seeds, dried fruits, and dark chocolate for a satisfying treat.
100. Make your own popcorn with olive oil and a sprinkle of nutritional yeast for a light and tasty snack.

Remember that individual nutritional needs vary, and it's important to create a balanced and diverse diet that meets your specific requirements. Consult a healthcare professional or registered dietitian before making significant changes to your diet, especially if you have underlying health conditions or dietary restrictions

Topical Treatments

Topical treatments, as a type of home remedy, involve the application of natural substances directly to the skin or external areas of the body to address various health concerns, promote healing, and provide relief from discomfort. These remedies make use of readily available ingredients that can be applied locally to the affected area. Topical treatments are particularly effective for skin issues, localized pain, and external discomforts. Here's a more detailed explanation:

External Application: Topical treatments are applied externally, targeting specific areas of the body where relief or healing is needed. This localized approach allows for direct contact with the affected area.

Skin-Focused Solutions: Topical treatments are commonly used to address skin-related concerns such as irritation, inflammation, dryness, rashes, and minor wounds. They can also offer cosmetic benefits by promoting healthy skin and enhancing its appearance.

Natural Ingredients: Many topical treatments are made from natural ingredients found in the kitchen, garden, or herbal pharmacy. Examples include herbs, essential oils, plant extracts, carrier oils, and other natural compounds.

Preparation Methods: Topical treatments can be prepared in various forms:

Salves and Balms: These are semi-solid mixtures containing herbal extracts, oils, and sometimes beeswax for consistency. They are convenient for direct application to the skin.

Ointments: Similar to salves, ointments have a softer consistency and often contain healing herbs infused in oils.

Creams and Lotions: These are water-based mixtures often containing herbal extracts and essential oils. They are absorbed quickly and can provide moisture to the skin.

Compresses and Poultices: These involve applying crushed or soaked herbs directly to the skin, often covered with a cloth to maintain contact.

Essential Oils: These concentrated plant extracts can be diluted with carrier oils and applied to the skin for specific benefits.

Common Uses: Topical treatments can be used for a variety of purposes, including:

Pain Relief: Applying analgesic herbs or essential oils to sore muscles or joints for pain relief.

Skin Irritations: Using soothing herbs or ingredients like aloe vera to calm irritated skin.

Wound Healing: Applying natural antiseptics like honey or calendula to minor cuts and wounds.

Skin Moisturizing: Using oils or creams to hydrate and nourish dry skin.

Anti-Inflammatory: Applying anti-inflammatory ingredients to reduce redness and swelling.

Bug Bites and Stings: Using soothing ingredients to relieve itching and discomfort.

Scar Reduction: Applying certain oils or herbal blends to promote the healing of scars.

Benefits and Considerations: Localized Action: Topical treatments provide targeted relief to specific areas, minimizing systemic effects.

Natural Approach: Many topical treatments avoid the use of synthetic chemicals, making them appealing to those seeking natural solutions.

Gentle and Non-Invasive: Topical remedies are generally non-invasive and can be suitable for sensitive individuals.

Professional Guidance: While topical treatments are generally safe, it's important to be cautious and seek guidance, especially if you have allergies or skin sensitivities.

Cautions and Safety: Some ingredients may cause allergic reactions or skin sensitivities, so patch testing is recommended.

Essential oils, in particular, should be diluted properly before application to avoid skin irritation. If you have a skin condition, open wound, or are pregnant, consult a healthcare professional before using topical treatments.

In summary, topical treatments offer a practical and targeted way to address external health concerns using natural ingredients. They can be part of a holistic approach to wellness, but it's important to exercise caution, perform patch tests, and consult with a healthcare professional if needed.

Here are 100 tips for using topical treatments as home remedies for various health and wellness concerns:

Skin Irritations and Healing:

1. Apply aloe vera gel to soothe sunburned skin.
2. Use calendula salve on minor cuts and scrapes for faster healing.
3. Dab honey onto a pimple to help reduce inflammation and promote healing.
4. Make a paste of turmeric and honey to address acne and blemishes.
5. Use coconut oil to moisturize and soothe dry, flaky skin.
6. Apply diluted chamomile essential oil to ease skin redness and irritation.
7. Create a cucumber mask to refresh and hydrate tired skin.
8. Use witch hazel as a natural astringent to tighten pores and reduce oiliness.
9. Mix oatmeal and yogurt to create a gentle exfoliating scrub for sensitive skin.
10. Apply diluted tea tree oil to help address fungal infections like athlete's foot.

Pain Relief:

11. Massage diluted lavender oil onto temples to ease tension headaches.
12. Create a ginger and cayenne pepper salve for muscle and joint pain relief.
13. Use arnica cream on bruises and sore muscles to promote healing.
14. Apply peppermint oil to temples and neck for headache relief.
15. Make a hot or cold compress using a cloth soaked in infused herbal tea for localized pain.
16. Use diluted eucalyptus oil in a massage oil for respiratory discomfort.
17. Apply diluted rosemary oil to ease muscle tension and promote circulation.
18. Use a warm mustard plaster on sore joints for relief.
19. Create a warm ginger compress for abdominal cramps and discomfort.
20. Apply diluted frankincense oil to alleviate arthritis pain and inflammation.

Skin Care and Beauty:

21. Massage jojoba oil onto your face as a natural makeup remover.
22. Create a honey and yogurt mask to cleanse and moisturize your skin.

23. Use diluted rose water as a toner to balance skin pH.
24. Apply diluted geranium oil to promote even skin tone and reduce scars.
25. Use a mixture of olive oil and sugar as a gentle lip scrub.
26. Apply diluted neroli oil to promote skin elasticity and reduce fine lines.
27. Make a baking soda and water paste to exfoliate and clarify your skin.
28. Use diluted carrot seed oil for its anti-aging properties.
29. Apply a slice of potato to dark under-eye circles to reduce puffiness.
30. Use diluted myrrh oil to address chapped and cracked skin.

First Aid and Minor Wounds:

31. Apply crushed plantain leaves to insect bites and stings for itch relief.
32. Use diluted lavender oil on minor burns to soothe pain and promote healing.
33. Apply a paste of baking soda and water to alleviate bee stings.
34. Create a poultice of crushed garlic and olive oil for ear infections.
35. Apply crushed fresh parsley to alleviate bruises.
36. Use diluted helichrysum oil on cuts and wounds to prevent infection.
37. Apply diluted chamomile oil to ease skin irritation from rashes.
38. Make a paste of turmeric and coconut oil to promote wound healing.
39. Apply diluted tea tree oil to small cuts and scrapes as a natural antiseptic.
40. Use aloe vera gel on minor burns and scalds for soothing relief.

Nail and Foot Care:

41. Soak your feet in warm water with Epsom salt to relieve foot pain.
42. Apply diluted lemon oil to strengthen brittle nails.
43. Use a mixture of tea tree oil and coconut oil to address toenail fungus.
44. Soak your feet in warm water with apple cider vinegar to soften calluses.
45. Apply diluted lavender oil to soothe tired feet and improve circulation.
46. Make a foot scrub using salt and olive oil to exfoliate rough skin.
47. Use diluted oregano oil for its antifungal properties on toenail infections.
48. Apply shea butter to moisturize dry cuticles and nails.
49. Mix baking soda and water to create a foot soak for odor control.
50. Apply diluted peppermint oil to refresh and cool tired feet.

Hair and Scalp Health:

51. Massage coconut oil into your scalp to moisturize and promote hair growth.

52. Apply diluted rosemary oil to address dandruff and improve scalp health.
53. Create an egg and yogurt mask to nourish and strengthen hair.
54. Use diluted chamomile oil to soothe an itchy scalp.
55. Apply aloe vera gel to soothe scalp irritation and inflammation.
56. Use diluted tea tree oil to address scalp conditions like lice.
57. Apply diluted lavender oil to calm frizzy hair and promote shine.
58. Create a hair mask with honey and olive oil for added moisture.
59. Use diluted peppermint oil to stimulate hair follicles and promote circulation.
60. Apply diluted cedarwood oil to support a healthy scalp and reduce hair loss.

Lip Care:

61. Apply a honey and sugar scrub to exfoliate chapped lips.
62. Use coconut oil to moisturize dry and cracked lips.
63. Apply a slice of cucumber to soothe and hydrate chapped lips.
64. Create a lip balm with beeswax, shea butter, and essential oils.
65. Use a mixture of honey and lemon juice to lighten dark lips.
66. Apply a thin layer of aloe vera gel to soothe sunburned lips.
67. Use cocoa butter to nourish and protect your lips from the elements.
68. Apply diluted chamomile oil to calm irritated and sensitive lips.
69. Create a lip mask with yogurt and honey to moisturize and soften lips.
70. Use rosehip oil to promote healing and reduce scarring on lips.

Hydration and Moisturization:

71. Apply coconut oil to your skin after a shower for all-over moisturization.
72. Use shea butter to deeply moisturize dry and rough skin areas.
73. Apply a thin layer of honey to your face for natural hydration.
74. Create a hydrating face mask with mashed avocado and yogurt.
75. Use aloe vera gel to soothe and moisturize sun-exposed skin.
76. Apply jojoba oil to your body to lock in moisture.
77. Create a nourishing body butter with cocoa butter and almond oil.
78. Use argan oil as a lightweight and non-greasy moisturizer for face and body.
79. Apply diluted lavender oil to moisturize and soothe dry, irritated skin.
80. Use rose water as a refreshing and hydrating facial mist.

Bug Bites and Stings:

81. Apply diluted peppermint oil to mosquito bites for cooling relief.
82. Use a slice of onion to alleviate itching from insect bites.
83. Create a paste of baking soda and water to soothe bee stings.
84. Apply aloe vera gel to soothe and calm skin after bug bites.
85. Use diluted tea tree oil on bug bites to prevent infection and reduce swelling.
86. Apply diluted eucalyptus oil to deter insects and soothe bites.
87. Use a mixture of apple cider vinegar and water to relieve itching from bites.
88. Create a paste of activated charcoal and water to draw out toxins from stings.
89. Apply crushed basil leaves to mosquito bites for natural relief.
90. Use a cold compress to alleviate itching and redness from insect bites.

Sensitive Skin Care:

91. Apply diluted chamomile oil to calm and soothe sensitive skin.
92. Use colloidal oatmeal in a bath to relieve itching and irritation.
93. Create a gentle face mask with yogurt and honey for sensitive skin.
94. Apply cucumber slices to soothe and hydrate sensitive skin areas.
95. Use calendula-infused oil to promote healing and reduce inflammation.
96. Apply aloe vera gel to soothe and cool irritated skin.
97. Use diluted rose water as a calming and hydrating facial toner.
98. Apply a mixture of coconut oil and shea butter to sensitive skin patches.
99. Create a fragrance-free lotion with natural moisturizers like cocoa butter and almond oil.
100. Use diluted lavender oil for its gentle and soothing effects on sensitive skin.

Remember that everyone's skin is unique, so it's important to perform patch tests when using new ingredients and consult a healthcare professional or dermatologist if you have specific skin concerns or sensitivities.

Inhalation Therapy

Inhalation therapy, also known as respiratory or inhalation remedies, is a type of home remedy that involves the inhalation of natural substances or vapors to promote respiratory health, alleviate congestion, and provide relief from various respiratory symptoms. This therapy focuses on delivering therapeutic compounds directly to the respiratory system through inhalation, which can have beneficial effects on the lungs, airways, and overall respiratory function. Inhalation therapy can be effective for addressing issues such as congestion, cough, sinusitis, and other respiratory discomforts. Here's a more detailed explanation:

Direct Delivery to the Respiratory System: Inhalation therapy offers a direct way to deliver natural compounds to the respiratory system. When inhaled, the therapeutic substances come into direct contact with the mucous membranes, airways, and lungs, providing rapid relief and targeted action.

Types of Inhalation: There are several methods of inhalation therapy, each utilizing different techniques to deliver therapeutic vapors or particles:

Steam Inhalation: Inhaling steam infused with essential oils or herbal extracts.

Aromatherapy Diffusion: Using essential oil diffusers to disperse aromatic molecules into the air.

Nebulizers: Devices that convert liquid solutions into fine mist for inhalation.

Inhalers: Portable devices containing essential oils or herbal blends for on-the-go use.

Hot Towel Inhalation: Placing a hot, damp towel infused with essential oils over the face to inhale the vapors.

Direct Inhalation: Inhaling the aroma of essential oils from a bottle or tissue.

Common Uses: Inhalation therapy is often used to address a range of respiratory concerns, including:

Congestion: Inhaling steam or essential oil vapors can help clear nasal passages and reduce congestion.

Cough: Certain inhalants, like eucalyptus or peppermint, can soothe cough and support respiratory comfort.

Sinusitis: Steam inhalation with eucalyptus or tea tree oil can help alleviate sinus congestion and pain.

Bronchitis: Inhalation of essential oils like thyme or frankincense can provide relief from bronchial discomfort.

Allergies: Inhaling chamomile or lavender can help calm allergy-related respiratory symptoms.

Stress and Relaxation: Aromatherapy diffusion with calming essential oils can promote relaxation and ease stress, indirectly benefiting respiratory function.

Beneficial Compounds: The therapeutic compounds used in inhalation therapy can include:

Essential Oils: These concentrated plant extracts contain aromatic molecules with various health benefits.

Herbal Extracts: Herbal remedies like chamomile, eucalyptus, and thyme are often used in steam inhalation.

Hydrosols: These are aromatic waters produced during the steam distillation of plants and can be used in diffusion.

Carrier Oils: Essential oils are often diluted in carrier oils for safe inhalation.

Safety Considerations:

Essential oils should be used with caution and properly diluted to prevent skin or respiratory irritation.

Inhalation therapy should not replace medical treatment for severe respiratory conditions.

People with respiratory conditions like asthma or allergies should consult a healthcare professional before using inhalation therapy.

Convenience and Accessibility: Inhalation therapy is convenient and can be done at home, making it easily accessible for self-care and immediate relief.

Inhalation therapy is a type of home remedy that involves inhaling natural substances, such as essential oils or herbal vapors, to support respiratory health and provide relief from respiratory discomfort. It offers a targeted and effective way to address various respiratory symptoms and promote overall well-being. However, it's important to use inhalation therapy with care, following proper guidelines and consulting a healthcare professional if you have specific health concerns or conditions.

Here are 20 tips for using inhalation therapy as a home remedy for various respiratory concerns and overall well-being:

1. Steam Inhalation:

Boil water and pour it into a bowl.

Add a few drops of eucalyptus essential oil to the hot water.

Lean over the bowl with a towel draped over your head and inhale the steam to relieve congestion.

For a calming effect, add lavender or chamomile essential oil to the steam.

Inhale steam for 5-10 minutes, taking breaks as needed.

2. Aromatherapy Diffusion:

Use an essential oil diffuser to disperse oils throughout the room.

Diffuse eucalyptus oil to clear the airways during cold and flu season.

Combine lavender and cedarwood oils for a soothing bedtime blend.

Diffuse peppermint oil to promote alertness and ease respiratory discomfort.

Experiment with different essential oil blends to find your preferred aromas.

3. Nebulizers:

Use a nebulizer to create a fine mist of essential oils for deep inhalation.

Inhale nebulized chamomile oil to alleviate allergy symptoms.

Nebulize tea tree oil to address sinus congestion and infection.

Combine lemon and lavender oils for a refreshing and cleansing inhalation.

Follow the manufacturer's instructions for proper nebulizer use.

4.   Inhalers:

Carry a personal inhaler with you for on-the-go relief.

Use a blend of peppermint and eucalyptus oils in your inhaler for respiratory support.

Inhale lavender oil from your inhaler to reduce stress and anxiety.

Customize inhaler blends for specific needs, such as focus or relaxation.

Replace the wick in your inhaler when the aroma diminishes.

5.   Hot Towel Inhalation:

Soak a small towel in hot water and wring it out.

Add a few drops of your chosen essential oil to the damp towel.

Place the warm, aromatic towel over your face and inhale deeply.

Use this method before bedtime with lavender oil for a restful sleep.

Relax with a hot towel inhalation session during your self-care routine.

6.   Direct Inhalation:

Inhale the scent of a calming essential oil like lavender directly from the bottle.

Carry a small vial of peppermint oil for a quick energy boost.

Inhale eucalyptus oil to clear your sinuses when you have a cold.

Directly inhale a citrus oil like orange or lemon for a mood uplift.

Keep a few inhalation oils in your purse or pocket for easy access.

7.Allergy Relief:

Diffuse a blend of lavender, lemon, and peppermint oils to ease allergy symptoms.

Inhale chamomile oil to calm allergic reactions and reduce inflammation.

Use steam inhalation with eucalyptus oil to clear nasal passages during allergy season.

Create a personalized allergy inhaler with oils that work best for you.

Keep inhalation oils on hand to address sudden allergy flare-ups.

8.   Respiratory Comfort:\

Use eucalyptus oil in a diffuser or steam inhalation to alleviate respiratory discomfort.

Nebulize a blend of tea tree and lavender oils for respiratory support.

Inhale peppermint oil to ease breathing during a cold or flu.

Diffuse cedarwood oil to reduce congestion and promote better airflow.

Experiment with various inhalation methods to find what works best for your respiratory needs.

9. Stress Reduction:

Inhale lavender or bergamot oil to reduce stress and anxiety.

Create a relaxation blend with frankincense and ylang-ylang for deep inhalation.

Use hot towel inhalation with a calming oil before bedtime for relaxation.

Diffuse a soothing essential oil blend in your bedroom to promote restful sleep.

Keep a stress-relief inhaler in your desk or bag for quick relaxation breaks.

10. Focus and Alertness:

Inhale rosemary or peppermint oil to boost focus and mental clarity.

Create an invigorating inhalation blend with lemon and ginger oils.

Use an inhaler with uplifting oils like citrus or eucalyptus during work or study sessions.

Diffuse essential oils known for their cognitive benefits, such as basil or rosemary.

Inhale a focus-enhancing blend before tasks that require concentration.

11. Emotional Balance:

Inhale lavender or chamomile oil to ease feelings of anxiety.

Create a comforting inhaler blend with cedarwood and vanilla oils.

Use hot towel inhalation with your favorite soothing oil during moments of emotional stress.

Diffuse a calming blend of essential oils in your living space.

Keep an emotional support inhaler on hand for grounding during challenging times.

12. Children and Inhalation:

For children, use gentle oils like lavender or chamomile for inhalation.

Create a kid-friendly inhaler with a diluted blend of calming oils.

Supervise children when using steam inhalation and ensure it's not too hot.

Use diffusion with mild oils like citrus or lavender in children's bedrooms for relaxation.

Consult with a pediatrician or aromatherapist for safe inhalation options for kids.

13. Throat and Cough Relief:

Inhale steam infused with tea tree or eucalyptus oil to soothe a sore throat.

Diffuse a throat relief blend with oils like peppermint and ginger.

Use a personal inhaler with a cough-calming blend during the day.

Inhale steam with thyme oil to support respiratory comfort.

Keep inhalation oils on hand for quick throat and cough relief.

14. Sinus Congestion:

Inhale steam with peppermint or eucalyptus oil to clear sinus congestion.

Diffuse a sinus relief blend with oils like rosemary and lemon.

Use a steam inhalation method with tea tree oil to address sinusitis.

Create a sinus inhaler with oils that help reduce congestion.

Keep inhalation remedies in your bathroom for sinus relief during showers.

15. Travel and Motion Sickness:

Inhale ginger oil to ease motion sickness during travel.

Create a portable inhaler with oils like peppermint for on-the-go relief.

Use steam inhalation with ginger oil before traveling to prevent nausea.

Inhale a blend of citrus and mint oils to combat travel fatigue.

Keep travel inhalation remedies in your travel bag or car.

16. Seasonal Support:

Inhale steam with lavender or chamomile oil to ease stress during the holidays.

Diffuse a festive blend of essential oils during seasonal gatherings.

Create an immune-boosting inhalation blend with oils like clove and cinnamon.

Inhale a seasonal cheer blend with pine and citrus oils.

Keep inhalation remedies with seasonal scents to enhance holiday experiences.

17. Customized Inhalation:

Experiment with various essential oils to create personalized inhalation blends.

Adjust the number of drops based on your scent preferences and respiratory needs.

Create inhaler blends for different occasions, such as relaxation, focus, or sleep.

Combine complementary oils to achieve a well-rounded and effective inhalation blend.

Keep a journal to track the effects of different inhalation blends and methods.

18. Proper Dilution and Usage:

Dilute essential oils properly when creating inhalation blends.

Use carrier oils when creating inhalation blends for nebulizers or inhalers.

Follow recommended guidelines for the number of drops to use in different inhalation methods.

Be cautious with strong oils like cinnamon or oregano, and use sparingly in inhalation blends.

When in doubt, consult an aromatherapist or healthcare professional for proper usage.

19. Consultation and Precautions:

Consult a healthcare professional if you have underlying health conditions before using inhalation therapy.

Perform a patch test on your skin before inhaling a new essential oil to check for sensitivities.

Avoid inhalation therapy if you have respiratory allergies or sensitivities to strong scents.

Use inhalation therapy as a complementary approach, not a substitute for medical treatment.

Be mindful of the effects of different oils on your mood and well-being.

20. Environment and Equipment:

 Maintain a well-ventilated space when using inhalation therapy to prevent overwhelming aromas.

Clean your diffuser or nebulizer regularly to prevent oil buildup and maintain effectiveness.

Store inhalation oils in a cool, dark place to preserve their potency.

Keep inhalation remedies in various rooms for easy access when needed.

Enjoy the therapeutic benefits of inhalation therapy as part of your holistic self-care routine.

Remember that individual responses to essential oils and inhalation methods may vary. Start with small amounts, and if you experience any adverse reactions, discontinue use and consult a healthcare professional.

Dietary changes

Dietary changes, as a type of home remedy, involve making modifications to your daily eating habits and food choices to address health concerns, improve well-being, and support overall vitality. The foods you consume play a significant role in your health, and making thoughtful dietary changes can have a positive impact on various aspects of your physical and mental well-being. Here's a deeper look at dietary changes as a type of home remedy:

Nutritional Foundation: Dietary changes focus on using food as medicine by incorporating nutrient-dense foods that provide essential vitamins, minerals, antioxidants, and other bioactive compounds necessary for optimal health.

Specific Health Goals: Dietary changes can be tailored to address specific health goals, such as weight management, blood sugar control, heart health, digestion, immune support, and more.

Whole Foods Emphasis: The emphasis is on consuming whole foods in their natural state, such as fruits, vegetables, whole grains, lean proteins, nuts, seeds, and legumes.

Processed Foods Reduction: Reducing or eliminating highly processed foods, which are often high in added sugars, unhealthy fats, and artificial additives, is a common aspect of dietary changes.

Balanced Nutrition: Dietary changes aim to achieve a balanced intake of macronutrients (carbohydrates, proteins, and fats) and micronutrients (vitamins and minerals) to support overall health.

 Hydration Focus: Adequate hydration through water and hydrating foods is an important aspect of dietary changes for optimal bodily functions.

Gut Health Improvement: Certain dietary changes can promote a healthy gut microbiome, which is crucial for digestion, immunity, and overall well-being.

Inflammatory Response: Some dietary changes target reducing foods that contribute to inflammation, which is associated with various chronic diseases.

Antioxidant-Rich Foods: Including antioxidant-rich foods like berries, leafy greens, and colorful vegetables can help combat oxidative stress and support cellular health.

Fiber Intake: Dietary changes often involve increasing fiber intake through whole grains, fruits, vegetables, and legumes to support digestive health and promote a feeling of fullness.

Plant-Based Focus: Incorporating more plant-based foods and reducing animal products is a common approach in dietary changes for various health benefits.

Healthy Fats: Focusing on sources of healthy fats like avocados, nuts, seeds, and olive oil can contribute to heart health and overall well-being.

Mindful Eating: Practicing mindful eating, which involves paying attention to hunger cues, savoring flavors, and eating with intention, is often a component of dietary changes.

Individualized Approach: Dietary changes can be personalized based on factors such as age, gender, activity level, health status, and personal preferences.

Sustainable Lifestyle: Effective dietary changes are sustainable and fit into your lifestyle, ensuring that you can maintain them over the long term.

Examples of Dietary Changes for Specific Concerns:

Weight Management: Reducing portion sizes, increasing vegetable intake, focusing on lean proteins, and being mindful of calorie intake.

Heart Health: Incorporating more whole grains, omega-3 fatty acids, and reducing saturated and trans fats.

Blood Sugar Control: Choosing complex carbohydrates, monitoring sugar intake, and including high-fiber foods.

Digestive Health: Adding fiber-rich foods, fermented foods, and staying hydrated for proper digestion.

Inflammation Reduction: Emphasizing anti-inflammatory foods like turmeric, ginger, fatty fish, and berries.

Before making significant dietary changes, it's advisable to consult a healthcare professional or registered dietitian, especially if you have underlying health conditions or dietary restrictions. They can help you create a personalized plan that aligns with your health goals and individual needs.

Here are 100 tips for using dietary changes as a home remedy to promote health and well-being:

General Dietary Changes:

1. Gradually replace processed foods with whole, unprocessed options.

2. Focus on nutrient-dense foods like fruits, vegetables, lean proteins, and whole grains.
3. Read food labels to make informed choices about ingredients and nutritional content.
4. Cook more meals at home to have better control over ingredients.
5. Avoid sugary beverages and opt for water, herbal tea, or infused water.
6. Choose lean protein sources such as chicken, turkey, fish, and legumes.
7. Opt for complex carbohydrates like whole grains, sweet potatoes, and quinoa.
8. Reduce added salt by using herbs, spices, and citrus for flavor.
9. Prioritize fiber-rich foods to support digestion and satiety.
10. Eat a variety of colorful fruits and vegetables to ensure a range of nutrients.

Balanced Eating:

11. Aim for balanced meals that include protein, carbohydrates, and healthy fats.
12. Practice portion control by using smaller plates and being mindful of serving sizes.
13. Include protein-rich foods in each meal to stabilize blood sugar levels.
14. Enjoy healthy fats from sources like avocados, nuts, seeds, and olive oil.
15. Space meals and snacks evenly throughout the day to maintain energy levels.
16. Listen to your body's hunger and fullness cues and eat intuitively.

Mindful Eating:

17. Eat slowly and savor each bite to enhance the eating experience.
18. Avoid distractions like screens while eating to focus on your meal.
19. Engage your senses by appreciating the colors, textures, and flavors of your food.
20. Practice gratitude for the nourishment your food provides.

Hydration:

21. Drink water throughout the day to stay hydrated.
22. Start your morning with a glass of water to kickstart hydration.
23. Infuse water with fresh fruits, herbs, or cucumber slices for added flavor.
24. Limit sugary drinks like soda and choose water instead.

25. Carry a reusable water bottle to remind yourself to stay hydrated.

Vegetables and Fruits:

26. Fill half your plate with vegetables to ensure a variety of nutrients.
27. Experiment with different cooking methods for vegetables, such as roasting, steaming, or grilling.
28. Incorporate leafy greens like spinach, kale, and arugula into salads, smoothies, and dishes.
29. Snack on cut-up veggies with hummus or a yogurt-based dip.
30. Enjoy a variety of fresh, seasonal fruits as snacks or desserts.

Whole Grains:

31. Choose whole grain options like brown rice, quinoa, whole wheat pasta, and oats.
32. Replace refined grains with whole grain versions in recipes.
33. Add rolled oats to smoothies or use them to make overnight oats.
34. Experiment with ancient grains like farro, barley, and freekeh.
35. Use whole grain bread for sandwiches and toast.

Protein Sources:

36. Include plant-based protein sources like lentils, beans, chickpeas, and tofu.
37. Opt for lean cuts of meat and remove visible fat before cooking.
38. Try seafood options like salmon, sardines, and mackerel for omega-3 fatty acids.
39. Snack on nuts and seeds for a protein and healthy fat boost.
40. Incorporate eggs into your diet for a versatile protein source.

Healthy Fats:

41. Use olive oil for cooking and as a salad dressing.
42. Sprinkle flaxseeds, chia seeds, or walnuts on oatmeal or yogurt.
43. Include avocados in salads, sandwiches, and wraps for creamy texture and healthy fats.
44. Snack on a handful of almonds or pistachios for a satisfying crunch.
45. Cook with coconut oil for a tropical flavor in your dishes.

Dairy and Dairy Alternatives:

46. Choose low-fat or non-fat dairy options for milk, yogurt, and cheese.
47. Try plant-based milk alternatives like almond, soy, or oat milk.
48. Opt for plain yogurt and add your own fresh fruits and nuts for flavor.
49. Experiment with dairy-free yogurt options made from coconut or almond milk.
50. Use cheese in moderation and consider options with lower fat content.

Snacking and Desserts:

51. Opt for whole foods like fresh fruit, nuts, or cut vegetables for snacks.
52. Create your own trail mix with a mix of nuts, seeds, and dried fruits.
53. Bake your own healthier versions of cookies and muffins using whole grains and less sugar.
54. Choose dark chocolate with higher cocoa content for a treat.
55. Make a fruit salad with a variety of colorful fruits for a refreshing dessert.

Meal Planning and Preparation:

56. Plan your meals and snacks ahead of time to make healthier choices.
57. Batch cook meals to have nutritious options readily available.
58. Prep vegetables and fruits in advance for quick and easy meals.
59. Cook extra portions for dinner to have leftovers for lunch the next day.
60. Use herbs and spices to add flavor to dishes without relying on excessive salt or sugar.

Fiber Intake:

61. Include high-fiber foods like beans, lentils, whole grains, and vegetables in your diet.
62. Snack on fiber-rich foods like popcorn, whole fruit, or carrot sticks.
63. Add chia seeds or ground flaxseeds to smoothies or yogurt for an extra fiber boost.
64. Choose whole fruits over fruit juices to get the benefits of dietary fiber.
65. Aim for at least 25-30 grams of fiber per day for digestive health.

Limit Added Sugars:

66. Read ingredient labels to identify added sugars in packaged foods.

67. Reduce or eliminate sugary beverages like soda, energy drinks, and sweetened teas.
68. Use natural sweeteners like honey or maple syrup in moderation.
69. Satisfy your sweet tooth with naturally sweet foods like berries or dates.
70. Choose plain versions of yogurt and add your own sweeteners like honey or fruit.

Salt Reduction:

71. Use herbs, spices, and citrus to flavor your dishes instead of excessive salt.
72. Gradually reduce the amount of salt you add to recipes to adjust your taste preferences.
73. Choose low-sodium versions of packaged foods when available.
74. Rinse canned beans and vegetables to reduce sodium content.
75. Experiment with salt-free seasoning blends to enhance flavor.

Eating for Energy:

76. Include complex carbohydrates like whole grains and fruits to sustain energy levels.
77. Combine carbohydrates with protein and healthy fats to maintain balanced energy.
78. Avoid heavy meals that can lead to energy crashes and opt for lighter, balanced options.
79. Stay hydrated throughout the day to prevent dehydration-related fatigue.
80. Include snacks with a mix of protein, fiber, and healthy fats for sustained energy.

Bone Health:

81. Include calcium-rich foods like dairy, fortified plant-based milk, leafy greens, and almonds.
82. Choose vitamin D-fortified foods or spend time in sunlight for bone health.
83. Consume foods rich in magnesium, like nuts, seeds, spinach, and whole grains.
84. Incorporate vitamin K-rich foods like kale, broccoli, and Brussels sprouts.
85. Prioritize a well-balanced diet to support overall bone health.

Heart Health:

86. Choose lean protein sources like poultry, fish, beans, and legumes.
87. Include foods high in omega-3 fatty acids, such as fatty fish, walnuts, and flaxseeds.
88. Opt for whole grains to promote heart health and manage cholesterol levels.
89. Limit saturated and trans fats by choosing lean cuts of meat and healthy cooking oils.
90. Include fiber-rich foods to support heart health and maintain healthy cholesterol levels.

Immune Support:

91. Consume a variety of colorful fruits and vegetables rich in vitamins and antioxidants.
92. Include foods high in vitamin C, like citrus fruits, bell peppers, and strawberries.
93. Incorporate zinc-rich foods such as lean meats, nuts, seeds, and whole grains.
94. Choose probiotic-rich foods like yogurt, kefir, sauerkraut, and kimchi for gut health.
95. Prioritize a well-balanced diet to support overall immune function.

Digestive Health:

96. Consume high-fiber foods like beans, lentils, whole grains, and vegetables.
97. Include fermented foods like yogurt, kefir, and kimchi for probiotics.
98. Drink plenty of water and stay hydrated to support digestion.
99. Experiment with foods like ginger, peppermint, and fennel for digestive comfort.
100. Prioritize whole foods and avoid excessive processed foods to maintain a healthy gut.

Remember that dietary changes should be tailored to your individual needs, preferences, and health goals. Consulting with a registered dietitian or healthcare professional can provide personalized guidance and ensure that your dietary changes align with your specific requirements.

Hydrotherapy

Hydrotherapy, also known as water therapy, is a type of home remedy that involves using water in various forms and temperatures to promote health, relieve discomfort, and support healing. Hydrotherapy has been practiced for centuries in different cultures around the world, and it utilizes the natural properties of water to stimulate circulation, relax muscles, and encourage overall well-being. Here's a more detailed look at hydrotherapy as a type of home remedy:

Types of Hydrotherapy: Hydrotherapy encompasses a range of techniques, each involving the use of water in different ways. Some common forms of hydrotherapy include:

Hot Baths: Soaking in hot water to relax muscles, improve blood circulation, and relieve stress.

Cold Compresses: Applying cold water compresses to reduce inflammation, alleviate pain, and constrict blood vessels.

Contrast Baths: Alternating between hot and cold water applications to improve circulation and stimulate the immune system.

Steam Inhalation: Inhaling steam from hot water infused with herbs or essential oils to ease respiratory congestion.

Sitz Baths: Immersing the lower body in warm water to soothe conditions like hemorrhoids or postpartum discomfort.

Wet Wraps: Applying wet, warm cloths or bandages to specific body areas to relieve pain or inflammation.

Foot Baths: Soaking the feet in warm water to relax the entire body, improve circulation, and soothe tired feet.

Circulatory Stimulation: Hydrotherapy can help improve blood circulation by alternately dilating and constricting blood vessels through hot and cold water applications. This can aid in detoxification and nutrient delivery to cells.

Muscle Relaxation: Hot water soaks and baths can relax muscles, alleviate tension, and promote a sense of relaxation. Cold water applications can also reduce muscle inflammation and soreness.

Pain Relief: Cold compresses and contrast baths can alleviate pain and reduce inflammation in sore or injured areas of the body.

Immune System Support: Alternating between hot and cold water applications, as in contrast baths, can stimulate the immune system and enhance its response.

Stress Reduction: Soaking in a warm bath or practicing hydrotherapy techniques can help reduce stress, promote relaxation, and improve mood.

Digestive Health: Hydrotherapy techniques like warm compresses or abdominal applications can promote healthy digestion and alleviate gastrointestinal discomfort.

Respiratory Relief: Steam inhalation can help open respiratory passages, ease congestion, and soothe irritation in the airways.

Skin Health: Hydrotherapy can improve skin circulation and may aid in detoxification, promoting a healthy complexion.

Lymphatic System Support: Hydrotherapy techniques that involve temperature variations can support lymphatic circulation, which helps remove waste and toxins from the body.

Safety and Precautions:

Consult a healthcare professional before trying hydrotherapy, especially if you have underlying health conditions.

Ensure that water temperatures are safe and comfortable, avoiding extremes that could cause burns or chills.

Be cautious with hydrotherapy if you have cardiovascular conditions, diabetes, or other medical issues.

Pay attention to your body's response and discontinue if you experience discomfort, dizziness, or other adverse effects.

Hydrotherapy at Home:

For a hot bath, run a comfortably warm bath and add Epsom salts, essential oils, or herbs for added relaxation.

Try alternating between a warm bath and a cool shower to experience the benefits of contrast hydrotherapy.

Use a cold compress or ice pack wrapped in a cloth to reduce swelling and ease pain.

Practice steam inhalation by adding a few drops of essential oil to a bowl of hot water, placing a towel over your head, and inhaling the steam.

Create your own foot soak by adding Epsom salts and a few drops of lavender oil to warm water.

Hydrotherapy is generally safe when practiced mindfully, but it's essential to listen to your body and consult a healthcare professional if you have concerns or medical conditions.

100 tips for using hydrotherapy as a home remedy to promote relaxation, relieve discomfort, and support overall well-being:

Hot Water Techniques:

1. Take a relaxing hot bath with Epsom salts to soothe muscles and unwind.
2. Add a few drops of lavender or chamomile essential oil to your bath for aromatherapy relaxation.
3. Use a warm compress on sore muscles to alleviate tension.
4. Place a warm, damp cloth over your eyes to soothe headaches and eye strain.
5. Enjoy a cup of herbal tea while soaking in a warm bath for a soothing experience.

Cold Water Techniques:

6. Apply a cold compress to reduce inflammation and pain in swollen areas.
7. Use a cold pack wrapped in a thin cloth on the forehead to ease headaches.
8. Dip your feet in cold water to help cool down on a hot day.
9. Splash your face with cold water in the morning to invigorate your skin and senses.
10. Take a cold shower to boost alertness and circulation.

Contrast Hydrotherapy:

11. Alternate between hot and cold water in the shower for an invigorating start to your day.
12. Try contrast baths by soaking your feet or hands in alternating hot and cold water.
13. Use a warm cloth followed by a cold cloth on your forehead to alleviate sinus congestion.
14. Alternate hot and cold compresses on sore muscles to stimulate circulation.
15. Practice contrast hydrotherapy by switching between a warm soak and a cool shower.

Steam Inhalation:

Add a few drops of eucalyptus or peppermint oil to hot water for steam inhalation to clear sinuses.

16. Inhale steam with lavender oil before bedtime to relax and promote restful sleep.
17. Use steam inhalation with chamomile oil to soothe respiratory discomfort.
18. Perform steam inhalation with tea tree oil to alleviate congestion and promote respiratory health.
19. Inhale the steam from a bowl of hot water infused with your favorite essential oil for relaxation.

Sitz Baths:

20. Take a warm sitz bath to soothe discomfort from hemorrhoids.
21. Add a few drops of witch hazel to your sitz bath water for added relief.
22. Consider using Epsom salts in your sitz bath to alleviate perineal discomfort after childbirth.
23. Perform a sitz bath with warm water infused with soothing herbs like calendula or chamomile.
24. Use a sitz bath to ease discomfort from vaginal irritation or postpartum healing.

Foot Baths:

25. Enjoy a warm foot soak with Epsom salts after a long day to relax tired feet.
26. Add a few drops of peppermint oil to a foot bath for a refreshing and cooling sensation.
27. Use a foot bath with warm water and lavender oil to relax before bedtime.
28. Try a cold foot soak to cool down during hot weather.
29. Create a soothing foot bath with warm water and a cup of chamomile tea.

Wet Wraps:

30. Apply a warm, damp cloth to sore joints to relieve pain and stiffness.
31. Use a cold, damp cloth on your forehead to reduce fever and discomfort.
32. Wrap a wet, warm cloth around your neck to alleviate neck tension.
33. Apply a warm, wet cloth to your chest to ease congestion during a cold.
34. Use a wet wrap on your abdomen with warm water to soothe digestive discomfort.

Hot and Cold Showers:

35. Start your shower with warm water to relax muscles, then gradually switch to cool water for circulation.
36. Alternate between hot and cold water in the shower to stimulate blood flow.
37. Begin your shower with warm water and end with a short burst of cold water to invigorate your senses.
38. Use a warm shower to relax before bed, followed by a cooler shower in the morning to wake up.

39. Try a contrast shower by alternating between 1 minute of hot water and 30 seconds of cold water.

Hydrotherapy for Relaxation:

40. Create a calming atmosphere by dimming the lights and playing soft music during your hydrotherapy session.
41. Practice deep breathing exercises while soaking in a warm bath to enhance relaxation.
42. Visualize stress melting away as you enjoy a warm soak or other hydrotherapy technique.
43. Combine hydrotherapy with mindfulness meditation for a holistic relaxation experience.
44. Use hydrotherapy as a regular part of your self-care routine to unwind and recharge.

Hydrotherapy for Sleep:

45. Take a warm bath infused with lavender or chamomile oil before bedtime to promote sleep.
46. Practice a warm foot soak with calming essential oils as part of your evening routine.
47. Perform steam inhalation with relaxing oils like lavender or bergamot before heading to bed.
48. Use a warm compress on your neck or shoulders to release tension and prepare for sleep.
49. Experiment with different hydrotherapy techniques to discover which ones help you sleep better.

Hydrotherapy for Muscle Relief:

50. Soak in a warm bath with Epsom salts after a strenuous workout to relax muscles.
51. Alternate hot and cold compresses on sore muscles to reduce inflammation and promote recovery.
52. Use a warm compress on your lower back to alleviate menstrual cramps.
53. Apply a cold compress to areas of pain or inflammation to numb and reduce discomfort.

54. Combine hydrotherapy with gentle stretching to enhance muscle relaxation and flexibility.

Hydrotherapy for Immune Support:

55. Use contrast showers to stimulate circulation and potentially boost immune function.
56. Enjoy steam inhalation with eucalyptus or tea tree oil to support respiratory health.
57. Take a warm bath with Epsom salts and a few drops of immune-boosting essential oils during cold and flu season.
58. Alternate between hot and cold compresses on your chest to support lymphatic circulation.
59. Incorporate hydrotherapy into your wellness routine to help maintain overall immune health.

Hydrotherapy for Skin Health:

60. Add oats or oatmeal to a warm bath to soothe itchy or irritated skin.
61. Use warm compresses to alleviate discomfort from insect bites or minor skin irritations.
62. Enjoy a gentle rain shower for a soothing experience that can enhance skin hydration.
63. Use hydrotherapy to complement your skincare routine by promoting blood flow and detoxification.
64. Combine hydrotherapy with natural skincare products for a holistic approach to skin health.

Hydrotherapy for Stress Relief:

65. Practice deep breathing exercises while enjoying a warm bath to enhance relaxation.
66. Create a spa-like ambiance with scented candles and calming music during your hydrotherapy session.
67. Use hydrotherapy as a time to disconnect from screens and external distractions.
68. Incorporate mindfulness techniques, such as body scans, while practicing hydrotherapy for stress relief.

69. Make hydrotherapy a regular part of your self-care routine to reduce stress and promote well-being.

Hydrotherapy for Respiratory Comfort:

70. Enjoy steam inhalation with eucalyptus or peppermint oil to ease congestion and promote easier breathing.
71. Use a warm compress on your chest to alleviate discomfort from a persistent cough.
72. Try a warm foot soak with aromatic oils to help open nasal passages.
73. Take a warm bath to relax muscles and ease tension, which can be beneficial for respiratory comfort.
74. Experiment with hydrotherapy techniques to find those that provide relief for your respiratory symptoms.

Hydrotherapy for Digestive Health:

75. Use a warm compress on your abdomen to relieve discomfort from gas or bloating.
76. Take a warm bath with calming essential oils to promote relaxation and ease digestive discomfort.
77. Enjoy a warm foot soak with ginger-infused water to support digestion.
78. Use hydrotherapy techniques in combination with mindful eating practices for optimal digestion.
79. Incorporate hydrotherapy as part of your digestive health routine to alleviate discomfort.

Hydrotherapy for Circulation:

80. Alternate between hot and cold water in the shower to stimulate blood flow and promote circulation.
81. Enjoy a warm bath with Epsom salts to help relax blood vessels and improve circulation.
82. Use hydrotherapy techniques in combination with gentle movement, like stretching or yoga, to enhance circulation.
83. Perform warm foot soaks with essential oils that have circulatory benefits, such as rosemary or cypress.
84. Make hydrotherapy a regular practice to support healthy blood circulation throughout the body.

Hydrotherapy for Joint Comfort:

85. Take a warm bath with Epsom salts to relax muscles and ease joint discomfort.
86. Alternate between warm and cold compresses on joints to reduce inflammation and promote relief.
87. Use hydrotherapy as a complement to your joint mobility exercises or physical therapy routine.
88. Enjoy a warm foot soak with relaxing essential oils to alleviate discomfort in your feet and ankles.
89. Experiment with different hydrotherapy techniques to find those that provide the most relief for your joints.

Hydrotherapy for Headaches:

90. Apply a cold compress to your forehead or the back of your neck to alleviate headache pain.
91. Use a warm compress on your forehead to relax tense muscles and potentially ease headache discomfort.
92. Combine hydrotherapy with relaxation techniques like deep breathing or meditation for headache relief.
93. Take a warm bath with calming essential oils to help relax and soothe headache symptoms.
94. Incorporate hydrotherapy into your headache management strategy for natural relief.

Hydrotherapy for Mood Enhancement:

95. Practice hydrotherapy techniques as a way to boost your mood and uplift your spirits.
96. Enjoy a warm bath with citrus-scented essential oils to promote a positive and energized mood.
97. Use hydrotherapy as a form of self-care to cultivate feelings of well-being and relaxation.
98. Alternate between warm and cool water in the shower to invigorate your senses and elevate your mood.
99. Make hydrotherapy a regular part of your routine to enhance your overall mood and emotional balance.

Remember to consider your individual preferences and any existing health conditions when practicing hydrotherapy. If you have specific health concerns or are unsure if hydrotherapy is suitable for you, consult a healthcare professional before incorporating these techniques into your wellness routine.

Lifestyle modifications

Lifestyle modifications, as a type of home remedy, involve making intentional changes to various aspects of your daily routine, habits, and behaviors to promote overall health, prevent health issues, and enhance your well-being. These modifications can encompass a wide range of areas, from physical activity and sleep to stress management and social interactions. Lifestyle changes are often a cornerstone of holistic health approaches and can have a profound impact on your quality of life. Here's a more detailed exploration of lifestyle modifications as a type of home remedy:

Physical Activity and Exercise: Regular physical activity can improve cardiovascular health, strengthen muscles, enhance flexibility, and contribute to weight management.

Incorporate a mix of aerobic exercises (walking, jogging, swimming) and strength training.

Engage in activities you enjoy to make exercise sustainable.

Set achievable fitness goals and gradually increase intensity over time.

Stay active throughout the day by taking short breaks from sitting and stretching.

Diet and Nutrition: Making mindful choices about what you eat can support overall health, energy levels, and immune function.

Focus on a balanced diet with a variety of nutrient-rich foods.

Prioritize whole foods like fruits, vegetables, whole grains, lean proteins, and healthy fats.

Control portion sizes to avoid overeating.

Limit added sugars, refined carbohydrates, and processed foods.

Stay hydrated by drinking water throughout the day.

Sleep and Rest: Quality sleep is essential for physical and mental well-being, as it allows the body to repair and rejuvenate.

Aim for 7-9 hours of restful sleep per night.

Establish a regular sleep schedule and maintain consistent bedtime and wake-up times.

Create a sleep-conducive environment by keeping your bedroom dark, quiet, and comfortable.

Limit screen time before bed to promote better sleep quality.

Stress Management: Managing stress effectively is crucial for maintaining emotional balance and preventing chronic health issues.

Practice relaxation techniques such as deep breathing, meditation, and mindfulness.

Engage in hobbies and activities that bring you joy and help you unwind.

Prioritize time for self-care and self-reflection.

Set realistic expectations and learn to say no when necessary.

Consider seeking support from friends, family, or professional counselors.

Mental and Emotional Well-being: Nurturing your mental health contributes to overall well-being and resilience.

Practice gratitude and positive self-talk.

Engage in activities that promote creativity and self-expression.

Cultivate healthy relationships and seek social connections.

Prioritize time for hobbies and interests that bring you happiness.

If needed, reach out to mental health professionals for guidance and support.

Smoking Cessation and Substance Use: Quitting smoking and reducing or eliminating substance use can have significant health benefits.

Seek resources and support to quit smoking or using tobacco products.

If you consume alcohol, do so in moderation and be mindful of its effects on your health.

Time Management and Organization: Effective time management and organization can reduce stress and improve productivity.

Use tools like calendars and to-do lists to prioritize tasks.

Break larger tasks into smaller, manageable steps.

Delegate tasks when possible to avoid feeling overwhelmed.

Social Connections: Building and maintaining social relationships can contribute to emotional well-being and provide a support network.

Spend quality time with family and friends.

Engage in group activities and social gatherings.

Foster connections through hobbies, clubs, or volunteer work.

Environmental Considerations: Creating a healthy living environment can positively impact your well-being.

Maintain a clean and organized living space.

Incorporate indoor plants to improve air quality and create a calming atmosphere.

Minimize exposure to environmental toxins.

Regular Health Check-ups: Regular medical check-ups and screenings can help identify potential health issues early and allow for timely interventions.

- Schedule routine visits to your healthcare provider.

- Follow recommended screenings based on your age, gender, and health history.

- Communicate openly with your healthcare provider about any health concerns.

Personal Development: Continuously seeking personal growth and learning can contribute to a sense of purpose and fulfillment.

- Set personal and professional goals to work toward.

- Engage in activities that challenge you and expand your skills.

- Embrace lifelong learning and explore new interests.

Mindful Technology Use: Mindful and intentional use of technology can prevent negative impacts on well-being.

- Set boundaries for screen time and digital device use.

- Prioritize face-to-face interactions over virtual ones.

- Engage in digital detoxes by taking breaks from screens.

Lifestyle modifications are a holistic approach to well-being that require commitment, patience, and ongoing effort. They can be personalized to suit your individual preferences, needs, and goals. Consulting with healthcare professionals, such as doctors, nutritionists, or therapists, can provide tailored guidance and support in making effective lifestyle changes.

100 tips for using lifestyle modifications as a type of home remedy to improve your overall health and well-being:

Physical Activity and Exercise:

1. Set a goal to engage in at least 30 minutes of moderate exercise most days of the week.

2. Choose physical activities that you enjoy to make exercise more sustainable.
3. Incorporate stretching or yoga to improve flexibility and prevent muscle stiffness.
4. Find an exercise buddy to make workouts more enjoyable and keep each other motivated.
5. Use a fitness tracker or app to monitor your progress and set achievable goals.

Diet and Nutrition:

6. Plan and prepare your meals in advance to make healthier choices.
7. Practice mindful eating by savoring each bite and paying attention to hunger cues.
8. Opt for smaller, more frequent meals to maintain stable energy levels throughout the day.
9. Experiment with new recipes to add variety and excitement to your diet.
10. Keep a food journal to track your eating habits and identify areas for improvement.

Sleep and Rest:

11. Establish a regular sleep schedule by going to bed and waking up at the same times each day.
12. Create a relaxing bedtime routine to signal to your body that it's time to wind down.
13. Make your sleep environment comfortable and conducive to rest.
14. Limit caffeine intake, especially in the afternoon and evening, to improve sleep quality.
15. Avoid heavy meals and excessive fluids close to bedtime to prevent disruptions.

Stress Management:

16. Practice deep breathing exercises to reduce stress and calm your mind.
17. Dedicate time to hobbies and activities that bring you joy and relaxation.
18. Try progressive muscle relaxation to release tension in your body.
19. Set aside time for mindfulness meditation to stay present and manage stress.

20. Incorporate breaks throughout your day to recharge and refocus.

Mental and Emotional Well-being:

21. Practice gratitude by listing things you're thankful for each day.
22. Engage in activities that promote creativity and self-expression, like drawing or journaling.
23. Reach out to friends and family to maintain social connections and emotional support.
24. Take breaks from screens and spend time outdoors to improve your mood.
25. Consider practicing daily affirmations to cultivate a positive self-image.

Smoking Cessation and Substance Use:

26. Seek resources and support to quit smoking or using tobacco products.
27. Identify triggers for substance use and find healthier alternatives to cope.
28. Create a plan for managing cravings and staying committed to quitting.
29. Engage in activities that keep your hands and mind busy to distract from cravings.
30. Celebrate small victories along your journey to quitting.

Time Management and Organization:

31. Use time-blocking to schedule specific tasks and prioritize your day.
32. Break larger tasks into smaller, manageable steps to avoid feeling overwhelmed.
33. Declutter your physical and digital spaces for a more organized environment.
34. Delegate tasks when possible to prevent burnout and improve efficiency.
35. Practice the "two-minute rule" to tackle quick tasks immediately and prevent procrastination.

Social Connections:

36. Reach out to friends and family regularly through phone calls, video chats, or in-person meetings.
37. Participate in group activities or join clubs that align with your interests.
38. Offer your support and lend a listening ear to others to strengthen relationships.
39. Attend social events, even if virtually, to maintain a sense of belonging.

Environmental Considerations:

40. Prioritize quality time with loved ones to foster meaningful connections.
41. Keep your living space clean and clutter-free for a sense of calm and order.
42. Incorporate indoor plants to improve air quality and create a soothing atmosphere.
43. Opt for natural light whenever possible to enhance your living environment.
44. Use calming colors in your decor to create a relaxing ambiance.
45. Use natural and non-toxic cleaning products to promote a healthier living space.

Regular Health Check-ups:

46. Schedule routine visits to your healthcare provider for preventive screenings and assessments.
47. Keep track of your health records, medications, and vaccinations in an organized manner.
48. Discuss your health concerns openly with your healthcare provider for personalized advice.
49. Stay up-to-date with age-appropriate screenings and vaccinations to catch health issues early.
50. Keep a journal of your symptoms and health-related questions to discuss during appointments.

Personal Development:

51. Set both short-term and long-term personal and professional goals.
52. Attend workshops, seminars, or online courses to expand your skills and knowledge.
53. Step out of your comfort zone and embrace new challenges to promote personal growth.
54. Reflect on your achievements and learn from setbacks to foster resilience.
55. Surround yourself with individuals who inspire and support your personal development.

Mindful Technology Use:

56. Set limits on screen time to prevent excessive use of digital devices.

57. Establish screen-free zones or times to promote face-to-face interactions.
58. Use productivity apps to help manage your time and digital distractions.
59. Disable notifications during designated periods to reduce interruptions.
60. Practice digital detoxes by taking breaks from screens and engaging in offline activities.

Nutritional Supplements and Vitamins:

61. Consult a healthcare professional before adding supplements to your routine.
62. Choose high-quality supplements from reputable brands to ensure effectiveness and safety.
63. Consider supplements that complement your dietary needs, such as vitamin D or omega-3 fatty acids.
64. Follow recommended dosages and guidelines provided by your healthcare provider.
65. Monitor how supplements affect your body and adjust your routine as needed.

Hydration:

66. Carry a reusable water bottle with you to remind yourself to stay hydrated.
67. Set reminders to drink water throughout the day, especially if you have a busy schedule.
68. Infuse water with fresh fruits, herbs, or cucumber slices for added flavor.
69. Consume hydrating foods like watermelon, cucumbers, and leafy greens.
70. Limit sugary beverages and opt for water, herbal tea, or infused water instead.

Mindful Eating:

71. Practice mindful eating by savoring each bite and eating slowly.
72. Eat when you're hungry and stop when you're comfortably satisfied.
73. Listen to your body's hunger and fullness cues to prevent overeating.
74. Avoid distractions while eating, such as screens or work, to focus on your meal.
75. Pay attention to the flavors, textures, and smells of your food to enhance your eating experience.

Meal Planning and Preparation:

76. Plan your meals and snacks ahead of time to make healthier choices.
77. Batch cook meals to have nutritious options readily available during busy days.
78. Prep fruits and vegetables in advance to streamline meal preparation.
79. Create a shopping list before grocery shopping to avoid impulse purchases.
80. Use versatile ingredients that can be used in multiple dishes to save time and reduce waste.

Mindful Cooking:

81. Choose whole and fresh ingredients for your recipes to prioritize nutrient intake.
82. Experiment with herbs and spices to enhance flavor without relying on excessive salt or sugar.
83. Explore different cooking methods like roasting, steaming, or sautéing for variety.
84. Involve family members in meal preparation to create bonding experiences.
85. Practice gratitude for the nourishment that food provides to your body.

Mindful Snacking:

86. Opt for nutrient-dense snacks like fresh fruits, vegetables, nuts, and seeds.
87. Portion out snacks to avoid mindless overeating from larger packages.
88. Choose snacks that provide a balance of protein, healthy fats, and fiber to keep you satisfied.
89. Avoid eating out of boredom or stress, and instead opt for mindful eating practices.
90. Practice intuitive eating by tuning in to your body's hunger and fullness signals.

Mealtime Rituals:

91. Create a calm and pleasant atmosphere for meals by dimming the lights and playing soft music.
92. Eat meals at a designated table or eating area to focus on your food.
93. Express gratitude for your meal before you begin eating.

94. Engage in conversation or self-reflection during meals to make them more mindful.
95. Chew your food thoroughly and enjoy the flavors and textures of each bite.

Balanced Eating Patterns:

96. Strive for balanced meals that include a combination of protein, complex carbohydrates, and healthy fats.
97. Include a variety of colorful fruits and vegetables to ensure a range of nutrients.
98. Aim to fill half your plate with vegetables, one-quarter with lean protein, and one-quarter with grains.
99. Limit highly processed and sugary foods, focusing on whole and minimally processed options.
100. Embrace a flexible approach to eating that allows for occasional treats while prioritizing nutrient-dense choices.

Remember, lifestyle modifications should be tailored to your individual needs, preferences, and health goals. Start by incorporating a few changes at a time and gradually build upon them. It's important to consult with healthcare professionals, such as doctors, registered dietitians, or fitness experts, to ensure that your lifestyle modifications are appropriate for your specific health situation.

Natural substances

Natural substances, as a type of home remedy, refer to using plant-based, herbal, and other naturally occurring materials to address various health concerns, promote wellness, and alleviate discomfort. These substances have been used for centuries in traditional medicine systems and are often sought after for their potential therapeutic benefits. From herbs and essential oils to natural remedies for skin care, natural substances offer a holistic approach to healing and well-being. Here's a more detailed exploration of using natural substances as a type of home remedy:

Herbal Remedies: Herbs are plant-based substances that have been used for their medicinal properties for generations. Herbal remedies involve using various parts of plants, such as leaves, roots, flowers, and seeds, to create infusions, teas, tinctures, and more. Some examples include:

Chamomile: Known for its calming properties, chamomile tea can help with relaxation and digestion.

Peppermint: Peppermint tea can aid in digestion and alleviate symptoms like bloating and indigestion.

Ginger: Often used to soothe nausea and improve digestion, ginger can be consumed as tea or added to meals.

Essential Oils: Essential oils are concentrated extracts from plants that capture their aromatic and therapeutic properties. They can be used in aromatherapy, massage, and topical applications. Examples include:

Lavender: Lavender oil is known for its calming effects and can be used for relaxation and sleep.

Tea Tree: Tea tree oil has antibacterial and antifungal properties, making it useful for skin issues.

Eucalyptus: Eucalyptus oil is commonly used for respiratory support and easing congestion.

Natural Oils: Natural oils derived from plants are often used in skincare and massage for their moisturizing and soothing properties. Examples include:

Coconut Oil: Known for its moisturizing effects, coconut oil can be used for skin and hair care.

Jojoba Oil: Jojoba oil is similar to skin's natural oils and is used for hydrating and balancing the skin.

Argan Oil: Rich in antioxidants, argan oil is used to nourish hair and improve skin health.

Honey and Propolis: Honey and propolis, a resin-like substance produced by bees, have been used for their potential antibacterial and wound-healing properties.

Honey: Raw honey can be used topically to promote wound healing and soothe sore throats.

Propolis: Propolis is used in natural remedies for its potential antimicrobial and immune-boosting properties.

Clay and Mud: Natural clays and mud have been used for skincare and detoxification purposes due to their mineral-rich composition.

Bentonite Clay: Often used in face masks, bentonite clay can help absorb excess oil and impurities.

Dead Sea Mud: Rich in minerals, Dead Sea mud is used for exfoliation and promoting healthy skin.

Apple Cider Vinegar: Apple cider vinegar is a fermented substance made from apples and is often used for its potential health benefits.

Digestive Aid: Diluted apple cider vinegar may aid digestion and alleviate symptoms like bloating.

Skin Care: It's sometimes used topically to balance the skin's pH and address skin concerns.

Aloe Vera: Aloe vera gel, extracted from the leaves of the aloe plant, is used for its soothing and cooling properties.

Skin Care: Aloe vera can be applied topically to soothe sunburns and promote skin healing.

Digestive Health: Some people use aloe vera juice for potential digestive benefits.

Natural Teas: Various herbal teas, such as nettle, dandelion, and hibiscus, are consumed for their potential health benefits.

Nettle Tea: Nettle tea is believed to support allergies and overall well-being.

Dandelion Tea: Dandelion tea may support liver health and act as a mild diuretic.

Hibiscus Tea: Hibiscus tea is rich in antioxidants and is often enjoyed for its tart flavor.

Turmeric and Curcumin: Turmeric is a spice known for its vibrant color and potential anti-inflammatory properties.

Golden Milk: A warm beverage made with turmeric, milk, and spices, often consumed for its potential health benefits.

Curcumin Supplements: Curcumin, the active compound in turmeric, is available in supplement form and is used for its potential anti-inflammatory effects.

Natural Sweeteners: - Stevia: A natural sweetener derived from the leaves of the stevia plant, it is used as a sugar substitute.

- Raw Honey: Raw honey is used as a natural sweetener and can contain enzymes and antioxidants.

These natural substances offer a holistic approach to health and well-being. However, it's important to note that while natural remedies have been used for generations, individual responses can vary, and not all remedies are supported by rigorous scientific research. Before using any natural substances for health purposes, it's advisable to do your research, consult with a healthcare professional, and ensure that they are safe and appropriate for your specific health condition.

100 tips for using natural substances as home remedies to promote health and well-being:

Herbal Remedies:

1. Brew a cup of chamomile tea to relax and unwind before bedtime.
2. Create a soothing lavender-infused oil for massages or to add to your bath.
3. Make a peppermint tea to ease digestive discomfort after a heavy meal.
4. Use ginger tea to soothe nausea and improve digestion.
5. Prepare a nettle tea for potential allergy relief and overall health.
6. Enjoy a cup of echinacea tea to support the immune system during cold and flu season.
7. Infuse thyme leaves in hot water for a homemade throat-soothing tea.
8. Brew a rosemary tea for potential cognitive benefits and improved focus.
9. Create an herbal steam inhalation with eucalyptus or thyme for respiratory relief.

10. Make a calendula-infused oil for soothing and healing skin irritations.

Essential Oils:

1. Diffuse lavender oil in your bedroom to promote relaxation and better sleep.
2. Add a few drops of tea tree oil to your shampoo to address scalp issues.
3. Use eucalyptus oil in a diffuser to ease congestion and promote clear breathing.
4. Apply diluted peppermint oil to your temples for headache relief.
5. Mix a calming blend of essential oils, like lavender and chamomile, for a relaxing massage oil.
6. Use diluted frankincense oil on your skin for potential anti-aging effects.
7. Inhale bergamot oil for mood upliftment and stress reduction.
8. Add a drop of lemon oil to your water for a refreshing and cleansing drink.
9. Apply diluted rosemary oil to your scalp to potentially promote hair growth.
10. Use a blend of essential oils in a warm bath for a spa-like experience.

Natural Oils:

1. Use coconut oil as a natural moisturizer for your skin and hair.
2. Apply jojoba oil to your face to balance oil production and hydrate the skin.
3. Massage argan oil onto split ends to nourish and repair damaged hair.
4. Create a natural lip balm using beeswax and coconut oil for soft lips.
5. Mix a few drops of rosehip oil into your moisturizer for added hydration.
6. Use avocado oil as a carrier oil for diluting essential oils for massage.
7. Apply almond oil to your cuticles to moisturize and promote healthy nails.
8. Use castor oil for a DIY eyelash and eyebrow growth serum.
9. Create a natural body scrub with olive oil and sugar for exfoliation.
10. Mix coconut oil with a few drops of tea tree oil for a natural deodorant.

Honey and Propolis:

1. Make a healing honey face mask by mixing raw honey with a splash of lemon juice.
2. Apply raw honey to minor cuts and wounds for its potential antibacterial properties.
3. Mix honey and cinnamon for a natural face scrub to promote glowing skin.

4. Create a honey-infused hair mask to condition and add shine to your hair.
5. Use honey to soothe a sore throat by adding it to warm water with lemon.
6. Apply propolis tincture to minor skin irritations for potential wound healing.
7. Make a DIY lip balm using beeswax, honey, and a touch of peppermint oil.
8. Mix honey and oats to create a gentle exfoliating facial cleanser.
9. Combine honey and yogurt for a hydrating and soothing face mask.
10. Make a honey and ginger tea for potential immune-boosting benefits.

Clay and Mud:

1. Create a bentonite clay face mask to draw out impurities and unclog pores.
2. Use Dead Sea mud as a body mask to exfoliate and nourish your skin.
3. Mix clay with water to create a poultice for insect bites and stings.
4. Apply a clay mask to your feet to refresh and detoxify after a long day.
5. Create a clay and rose water paste for a natural spot treatment for acne.
6. Use clay as an ingredient in a homemade toothpaste for potential teeth whitening.
7. Combine clay with herbal infusions for a custom hair mask.
8. Create a mud bath by adding Dead Sea mud to your bathwater for a spa experience.
9. Mix clay with water and a drop of lavender oil for a soothing face mask.
10. Apply a clay mask to your armpits as a natural detox for potential odor control.

Apple Cider Vinegar:

1. Dilute apple cider vinegar with water as a natural toner for your skin.
2. Create an apple cider vinegar hair rinse to clarify and promote shine.
3. Mix apple cider vinegar with water to use as a scalp clarifying treatment.
4. Add a tablespoon of apple cider vinegar to warm water as a morning detox drink.
5. Use apple cider vinegar as a natural cleaner for household surfaces.
6. Dilute apple cider vinegar with water and use it as a natural deodorant.
7. Soak your feet in a mixture of apple cider vinegar and warm water to soothe tired feet.
8. Mix apple cider vinegar with water to create a post-shampoo hair rinse for extra shine.

9. Combine apple cider vinegar with honey and water for a soothing throat gargle.
10. Add apple cider vinegar to your bathwater to help balance your skin's pH.

Aloe Vera:

1. Apply aloe vera gel to sunburned skin for soothing relief and hydration.
2. Use aloe vera gel as a natural makeup remover for gentle cleansing.
3. Create an aloe vera and cucumber face mask for cooling and hydrating the skin.
4. Apply aloe vera gel to minor cuts and abrasions to promote healing.
5. Mix aloe vera gel with a few drops of tea tree oil for a natural acne treatment.
6. Apply aloe vera gel to dry and itchy skin to alleviate discomfort.
7. Create a DIY after-sun lotion by mixing aloe vera gel with coconut oil.
8. Use aloe vera gel as a natural hair conditioner to hydrate and promote shine.
9. Make a soothing aloe vera and lavender oil body lotion for relaxation.
10. Mix aloe vera gel with rose water for a refreshing and calming facial mist.

Natural Teas:

1. Enjoy dandelion tea as a potential diuretic for detoxification.
2. Sip on hibiscus tea for its potential antioxidant and cardiovascular benefits.
3. Brew a cup of ginger tea to ease digestive discomfort and promote circulation.
4. Create a blend of chamomile and mint tea for relaxation and digestion.
5. Make a soothing licorice root tea for potential sore throat relief.
6. Drink green tea for its potential metabolism-boosting and antioxidant properties.
7. Enjoy a cup of lemon balm tea for relaxation and stress reduction.
8. Brew a cup of red clover tea for potential hormonal balance.
9. Create a blend of nettle and peppermint tea for potential allergy relief.
10. Make a calming valerian root tea to promote relaxation and better sleep.

Turmeric and Curcumin:

1. Add a pinch of turmeric to your smoothies for potential anti-inflammatory benefits.

2. Create a turmeric and honey face mask for a glowing complexion.
3. Mix turmeric with milk and honey for a soothing golden milk latte.
4. Use turmeric in cooking to add flavor and potential health benefits.
5. Make a DIY turmeric and yogurt mask to brighten and even out your skin tone.
6. Create a turmeric paste with coconut oil for potential wound healing.
7. Combine turmeric with water to create a natural toothpaste for oral health.
8. Mix turmeric and water to make a paste for spot treatment of acne.
9. Incorporate turmeric into your diet to potentially alleviate joint discomfort.
10. Take curcumin supplements after consulting with a healthcare professional.

Natural Sweeteners:

1. Use stevia as a natural sugar substitute in beverages and recipes.
2. Add raw honey to herbal teas for natural sweetness and potential health benefits.
3. Use maple syrup as a topping for pancakes, waffles, and desserts.
4. Incorporate coconut sugar as a natural alternative to refined sugar in baking.
5. Mix natural sweeteners with oats and nuts for a homemade granola.
6. Drizzle raw honey over yogurt and fresh fruit for a wholesome dessert.
7. Use date syrup as a natural sweetener in smoothies and baked goods.
8. Add a touch of natural sweetener to your morning coffee or tea.
9. Experiment with different natural sweeteners to find your favorites for various dishes.
10. Enjoy the flavors of natural sweeteners while being mindful of portion sizes.

When using natural substances as home remedies, always keep in mind that individual reactions may vary. It's important to do a patch test before applying any new substance to your skin, and consult with a healthcare professional before trying any new remedy, especially if you have allergies, sensitivities, or medical conditions.

Aromatherapy

Aromatherapy is a type of alternative medicine that involves using aromatic plant extracts, known as essential oils, to promote physical, mental, and emotional well-being. These essential oils are obtained from various parts of plants through methods like distillation or cold pressing, capturing their concentrated natural scents and therapeutic properties. Aromatherapy is commonly used for relaxation, stress relief, mood enhancement, and supporting overall health. Here's a more in-depth exploration of aromatherapy as a type of home remedy:

Essential Oils: Essential oils are the core of aromatherapy. They are highly concentrated plant extracts that contain the volatile compounds responsible for the unique scents and potential therapeutic effects of different plants. Each essential oil has its own set of properties and benefits, ranging from calming to energizing. Some commonly used essential oils include lavender, peppermint, eucalyptus, tea tree, chamomile, and lemon.

 Methods of Application: Aromatherapy offers various methods of application to enjoy the benefits of essential oils:

Diffusion: Using an aromatherapy diffuser, essential oils are dispersed into the air as fine mist, allowing you to inhale the aroma and experience its effects.

Topical Application: Diluted essential oils can be applied to the skin through massage, using carrier oils like coconut oil, jojoba oil, or almond oil. This allows the oils to be absorbed into the bloodstream.

Inhalation: Inhaling essential oils directly from the bottle, through a tissue, or by adding a few drops to hot water creates a direct effect on the respiratory system.

Baths: Adding a few drops of essential oils to a warm bath creates a soothing and aromatic experience.

Compresses: Applying a diluted essential oil mixture to a warm or cold compress and placing it on the skin provides localized relief.

Benefits of Aromatherapy:

Stress Reduction: Many essential oils have calming properties that can help reduce stress and anxiety. Lavender, chamomile, and bergamot are often used for relaxation.

Improved Sleep: Certain essential oils, such as lavender and cedarwood, are believed to promote better sleep and relaxation.

Mood Enhancement: Aromatherapy can uplift your mood and create a positive ambiance. Citrus oils like lemon and orange are known for their invigorating effects.

Pain Relief: Some essential oils, such as eucalyptus and peppermint, can be used topically to soothe muscle pain and headaches.

Respiratory Support: Eucalyptus, tea tree, and peppermint essential oils can help clear congested airways and provide relief from respiratory issues.

Skin Care: Essential oils like tea tree, lavender, and frankincense are often used for their potential benefits in promoting healthy skin.

Focus and Concentration: Essential oils like rosemary and peppermint may enhance alertness and focus.

Safety Considerations:

Essential oils are potent and should be used with caution. Always dilute them before applying to the skin, as some oils can cause skin irritation.

Some essential oils are not safe for pregnant women, infants, or certain medical conditions. Consult with a healthcare professional before using aromatherapy, especially in these cases.

Quality matters. Choose high-quality, pure essential oils from reputable sources to ensure their effectiveness and safety.

Creating an Aromatherapy Environment:

Choose an appropriate diffuser for your space. Ultrasonic diffusers are commonly used and offer a fine mist of essential oils into the air.

Experiment with different essential oil blends to find scents that resonate with you and provide the desired effects.

Practice mindfulness while enjoying aromatherapy. Take a moment to inhale deeply, allowing the aroma to envelop your senses.

Aromatherapy offers a versatile and enjoyable way to incorporate natural scents into your daily routine to support relaxation, wellness, and a balanced lifestyle.

100 tips for using aromatherapy as a type of home remedy to promote well-being and address various concerns:

Stress Reduction:

1. Diffuse lavender essential oil to create a calming atmosphere before bedtime.

2. Keep a roll-on bottle of a stress-relief blend (e.g., lavender, bergamot, and frankincense) to apply to your wrists and temples during stressful moments.

3. Add a few drops of chamomile essential oil to your evening bath for relaxation.

4. Carry a small inhaler with a calming blend to use when feeling anxious or stressed.

5. Place a few drops of cedarwood essential oil on a cotton ball and tuck it under your pillow for a peaceful night's sleep.

6. Create a calming room spray by mixing lavender and rose essential oils with water and spritzing your living space.

Sleep Improvement:

7. Diffuse a blend of lavender and cedarwood essential oils in your bedroom to aid sleep.

8. Use a pillow spray with lavender essential oil to promote restful sleep.

9. Apply a soothing blend of chamomile and marjoram essential oils to your pulse points before bedtime.

10. Create a bedtime routine that includes deep breathing with a calming essential oil like lavender.

11. Add a drop of vetiver essential oil to the soles of your feet for grounding and relaxation.

12. Inhale a blend of frankincense and bergamot essential oils to help ease nighttime restlessness.

Mood Enhancement:

13. Diffuse citrus essential oils like lemon, orange, or grapefruit to uplift your mood.

14. Carry a personal inhaler with a bright and energizing blend to use as a pick-me-up during the day.

15. Add a few drops of a mood-boosting blend to a tissue and inhale deeply when feeling down.

16. Create a mood-enhancing body lotion by adding your favorite uplifting essential oils to an unscented base.

17. Diffuse a blend of ylang-ylang and bergamot to create a romantic and positive atmosphere.

18. Use a citrusy essential oil blend in your morning shower for an invigorating start to the day.

Pain Relief:

19. Mix a few drops of peppermint essential oil with a carrier oil and massage it onto sore muscles.

20. Apply a warming blend of ginger and black pepper essential oils to soothe joint discomfort.

21. Use a roll-on bottle with a pain-relief blend for easy application to targeted areas.

22. Add a few drops of eucalyptus essential oil to a bowl of hot water for steam inhalation to relieve sinus congestion.

23. Create a soothing bath soak with lavender and marjoram essential oils for muscle relaxation.

24. Use a warming compress with a blend of rosemary and lavender essential oils to alleviate tension headaches.

Respiratory Support:

25. Inhale eucalyptus essential oil from a tissue to clear nasal congestion.

26. Use a chest rub with eucalyptus and tea tree oils for cough and cold relief.

27. Diffuse a blend of peppermint and eucalyptus to open up the airways during respiratory discomfort.

28. Make a DIY vapor rub with eucalyptus, peppermint, and coconut oil for chest congestion.

29. Add a few drops of frankincense essential oil to your steamy shower for potential respiratory benefits.

30. Create a soothing chest balm with eucalyptus and lemon essential oils for easy application.

Skin Care:

31. Dilute tea tree essential oil in a carrier oil and apply it to blemishes as a spot treatment.

32. Make a DIY facial steam with lavender and chamomile essential oils to cleanse and refresh your skin.

33. Add a drop of geranium essential oil to your moisturizer for potential skin-balancing benefits.

34. Mix lavender essential oil with aloe vera gel for a natural sunburn relief remedy.

35. Create a calming and hydrating facial mist with rose and chamomile essential oils.

36. Use a roll-on blend with lavender and tea tree essential oils for minor skin irritations.

Focus and Concentration:

37. Diffuse a blend of rosemary and lemon essential oils to enhance mental clarity.

38. Carry a focus-enhancing inhaler with you for use during work or study sessions.

39. Apply a roll-on blend with peppermint and rosemary essential oils to your wrists and temples for alertness.

40. Use a diffuser necklace with a concentration-enhancing essential oil blend.

41. Inhale a blend of basil and lemon essential oils when tackling challenging tasks.

42. Create a focus-promoting room spray with vetiver and cedarwood essential oils.

Digestive Health:

43. Dilute ginger essential oil in a carrier oil and massage it onto the abdomen for digestive relief.

44. Diffuse a blend of peppermint and fennel essential oils to alleviate indigestion.

45. Add a drop of lemon essential oil to a glass of water for potential digestive support.

46. Create a soothing belly rub with ginger and lavender essential oils for digestive discomfort.

47. Inhale a blend of cardamom and peppermint essential oils to ease nausea.

48. Use a digestion support roll-on blend for convenient application on the go.

Personal Care:

49. Add a few drops of your favorite essential oils to unscented shampoo or conditioner for a customized hair care experience.

50. Create a natural deodorant with baking soda, cornstarch, and essential oils like lavender and tea tree.

51. Make a refreshing mouthwash with peppermint and tea tree essential oils for oral hygiene.

52. Use a natural toothpaste recipe with baking soda and peppermint essential oil.

53. Create a luxurious body scrub with sugar, coconut oil, and essential oils for exfoliation.

54. Make a DIY perfume roller with your favorite essential oil blends for a personalized scent.

Aromatherapy for Children:

55. Use lavender essential oil in a diffuser to create a calming bedtime routine for children.

56. Dilute gentle essential oils like chamomile or mandarin in a carrier oil for children's massages.

57. Add a drop of lavender essential oil to a stuffed animal or pillow for comfort.

58. Create a kid-friendly inhaler with essential oils for focus and concentration during homework.

59. Diffuse a calming blend of essential oils in the playroom to create a peaceful environment.

60. Make a soothing bath soak with lavender and chamomile essential oils to relax before bedtime.

Seasonal Allergies:

61. Diffuse a blend of lavender, lemon, and peppermint essential oils for potential allergy relief.

62. Carry an allergy relief inhaler with you during allergy season.

63. Apply a roll-on blend with eucalyptus and tea tree oils to the chest and sinus areas.

64. Use a saline nasal spray with added essential oils to help clear nasal passages.

65. Create a soothing chest balm with lavender and eucalyptus oils for allergy-related discomfort.

66. Diffuse a blend of frankincense and myrrh essential oils to potentially support respiratory health.

Natural Cleaning:

67. Create a natural all-purpose cleaner with tea tree and lemon essential oils for disinfection.

68. Make a DIY citrus-infused vinegar cleaner with orange or grapefruit essential oil.

69. Use a lavender and lemon essential oil blend to freshen up linens and towels.

70. Diffuse cleansing essential oils like lemon and eucalyptus to purify the air in your home.

71. Create a natural air freshener with a blend of your favorite essential oils and water.

72. Add a few drops of essential oils to baking soda for a natural carpet deodorizer.

Emotional Well-Being:

73. Inhale a calming essential oil blend when practicing meditation or mindfulness.

74. Create a personalized aromatherapy roller with essential oils that resonate with your emotions.

75. Use a diffuser bracelet to carry your favorite emotional support essential oils with you.

76. Diffuse grounding essential oils like vetiver or patchouli to help center your emotions.

77. Inhale a blend of bergamot and frankincense essential oils to uplift your spirits.

78. Create an aroma blend to use during journaling or self-reflection sessions.

Special Occasions:

79. Diffuse festive essential oil blends during holiday gatherings for a cozy ambiance.

80. Create personalized essential oil blends as thoughtful gifts for friends and family.

81. Diffuse floral essential oils like rose and jasmine for a romantic and special atmosphere.

82. Add a few drops of a favorite essential oil to your DIY potpourri for fragrance.

83. Use an essential oil-infused candle during celebrations for an aromatic touch.

84. Create a calming essential oil blend to diffuse during yoga or relaxation sessions.

DIY Beauty Products:

85. Create a DIY facial oil with rosehip and geranium essential oils for glowing skin.

86. Mix a few drops of your favorite essential oils into your body lotion for a customized scent.

87. Make a nourishing hair serum with argan oil and ylang-ylang essential oil.

88. Add essential oils like lavender and cedarwood to your homemade bath bombs.

89. Create a refreshing body spray with essential oils and distilled water for a light scent.

90. Make a natural lip balm with beeswax, coconut oil, and peppermint essential oil.

Aromatherapy on the Go:

91. Use an essential oil inhaler while traveling to combat motion sickness.

92. Carry a personal inhaler with a blend of essential oils for stress relief during a busy day.

93. Apply an essential oil roll-on blend to your wrists before meetings or appointments.

94. Use a diffuser pendant to enjoy the benefits of aromatherapy throughout the day.

95. Create a travel-friendly essential oil first aid kit for minor discomforts.

96. Diffuse a grounding essential oil blend in your car to help stay focused during drives.

Mindful Rituals:

97. Incorporate aromatherapy into your morning or evening meditation practice.

98. Create an aromatherapy ritual before bedtime to wind down and relax.

99. Diffuse a blend of essential oils while practicing yoga for added focus and mindfulness.

100. Use aromatherapy as part of a gratitude practice, inhaling a calming blend while reflecting on positive aspects of your life.

When using aromatherapy, it's important to select high-quality, pure essential oils and practice safety guidelines, such as proper dilution and avoiding contact with sensitive areas like the eyes. Additionally, individual responses to essential oils can vary, so start with a small amount and observe how your body reacts. Always consult with a healthcare professional before using essential oils, especially if you have allergies, sensitivities, or underlying health conditions.

Physical manipulation

Physical manipulation as a type of home remedy involves using hands-on techniques to address various physical discomforts, improve mobility, and support overall well-being. These techniques are often employed to alleviate pain, enhance flexibility, and promote relaxation without the need for invasive procedures or medications. Here's a deeper look into physical manipulation as a home remedy:

Types of Physical Manipulation:

1. **Massage:** This involves applying pressure, kneading, and rubbing techniques to the body's soft tissues, such as muscles and fascia. Massaging can help relax muscles, reduce tension, and improve blood circulation.

2. **Stretching:** Gentle and controlled stretching exercises are used to lengthen muscles, improve flexibility, and maintain joint mobility.

3. **Joint Mobilization:** Through controlled movements, joint mobilization aims to restore proper joint function, reduce stiffness, and enhance range of motion.

4. **Self-Myofascial Release:** Techniques like foam rolling and using massage balls apply pressure to specific areas to release tension in muscles and fascia.

5. **Acupressure:** By applying pressure to specific points on the body, acupressure promotes relaxation, relieves pain, and supports energy flow.

6. **Spinal Manipulation:** Techniques like spinal twists and gentle adjustments aim to improve spinal alignment, alleviate back discomfort, and support nerve function.

7. **Breathing Exercises:** Certain breathing techniques, such as diaphragmatic breathing, promote relaxation, improve oxygenation, and reduce stress.

8. **Posture Correction:** Adjusting and maintaining proper posture helps prevent musculoskeletal issues and supports overall alignment.

Benefits of Physical Manipulation:

- **Pain Relief:** Physical manipulation can help reduce pain caused by muscle tension, stiffness, or minor injuries.

- **Improved Mobility:** Techniques like stretching and joint mobilization enhance flexibility and joint range of motion.

- **Stress Reduction:** Many manipulation techniques induce relaxation, leading to reduced stress and improved mood.

- **Enhanced Circulation:** Massaging and manipulating tissues improve blood flow, which aids in nutrient delivery and waste removal.

- **Injury Prevention:** Regular manipulation can help prevent injuries by maintaining joint health and muscle flexibility.

- **Muscle Recovery:** After physical activities, manipulation techniques can aid muscle recovery and alleviate soreness.

- **Nervous System Support:** Techniques like spinal manipulation may support nerve function and nervous system health.

Tips for Safe and Effective Physical Manipulation at Home:

1. **Educate Yourself:** Learn proper techniques from reliable sources, such as instructional videos, reputable websites, or certified instructors.

2. **Start Gently:** Begin with mild pressure and gentle movements, especially if you're new to manipulation techniques.

3. **Listen to Your Body:** Pay attention to your body's responses. If you experience pain or discomfort, stop the technique and seek professional guidance.

4. **Warm Up:** Always warm up your muscles before attempting stretching or manipulation to prevent injury.

5. **Stay Hydrated:** Proper hydration supports muscle health and overall well-being when practicing manipulation.

6. **Consistency Matters:** Regular practice yields better results. Incorporate manipulation techniques into your routine for ongoing benefits.

7. **Consult Professionals:** If you have chronic pain, injuries, or underlying health conditions, consult healthcare professionals or physical therapists before attempting manipulation.

8. **Use Props:** Tools like foam rollers, massage sticks, and resistance bands can enhance the effectiveness of your manipulation techniques.

9. **Incorporate Breathing:** Deep, mindful breathing can enhance the relaxation benefits of physical manipulation.

10. **Complement Other Remedies:** Physical manipulation can complement other home remedy types, such as hot/cold therapy, herbal remedies, and more.

Important Considerations:

- **Individual Variation:** Responses to manipulation vary. What works well for one person may not work the same for another.

- **Seek Professional Guidance:** For complex or chronic issues, consulting healthcare professionals or trained therapists is essential.

- **Caution with Certain Conditions:** Be cautious with conditions like herniated discs, osteoporosis, and recent injuries. Seek guidance before manipulation.

Physical manipulation as a home remedy offers a holistic and proactive approach to maintaining physical well-being. By incorporating these techniques into your routine, you can promote relaxation, improve mobility, and support your body's natural healing processes.

100 tips for using physical manipulation as a type of home remedy to address discomfort, enhance mobility, and support overall well-being:

Massage:

1. Use your fingertips to gently massage your temples to alleviate tension headaches.

2. Apply gentle pressure and circular motions to your neck and shoulders to release built-up tension.

3. Use a foam roller to roll along your back muscles to release knots and tightness.

4. Try self-massage on your feet using a tennis ball to promote relaxation and foot health.

5. Use long, sweeping strokes with a soft brush to stimulate circulation and exfoliate the skin.

6. Incorporate massage techniques during your daily skincare routine for facial relaxation.

Stretching:

7. Begin your day with a few minutes of gentle stretching to increase flexibility and energy.

8. Hold a standing calf stretch for 30 seconds on each leg to alleviate tightness.

9. Perform a seated spinal twist to release tension and improve spinal mobility.

10. Stretch your hip flexors by lunging forward and leaning slightly backward.

11. Incorporate yoga or Pilates routines that focus on flexibility and full-body stretching.

12. Perform neck stretches to relieve tension and improve neck mobility.

Joint Mobilization:

13. Gently rotate your wrists and ankles to maintain joint mobility and reduce stiffness.

14. Practice knee circles to enhance knee joint movement and reduce discomfort.

15. Perform shoulder rolls to improve shoulder joint flexibility and reduce tension.

16. Do gentle hip circles to promote hip joint mobility and reduce tightness.

17. Use a tennis ball to roll under your feet to promote foot joint health.

Self-Myofascial Release:

18. Roll a tennis ball under your feet to release tension and improve foot flexibility.

19. Use a foam roller to release tension in your quadriceps after a workout.

20. Roll a massage stick along your calf muscles to alleviate tightness.

21. Target the IT band by using a foam roller along the outer thigh area.

22. Use a foam roller to target your upper back and alleviate upper body tension.

Acupressure:

23. Apply gentle pressure to the space between your thumb and index finger to alleviate headaches.

24. Use acupressure on the inner wrist to help ease nausea and motion sickness.

25. Apply pressure to the base of your skull to potentially alleviate tension headaches.

26. Press the point between your eyebrows to promote relaxation and reduce stress.

27. Gently massage the area just below your kneecap to alleviate knee discomfort.

Spinal Manipulation:

28. Practice gentle spinal twists to improve spinal flexibility and alleviate back tension.

29. Do cat-cow stretches to promote spinal mobility and relieve lower back discomfort.

30. Perform a seated forward fold to stretch and align the spine.

31. Lie on your back and gently hug your knees to your chest to release lower back tension.

32. Incorporate gentle twists and stretches into your morning or evening routine.

Breathing Exercises:

33. Practice diaphragmatic breathing to reduce stress and promote relaxation.

34. Inhale deeply through your nose and exhale slowly through your mouth to calm your nervous system.

35. Use box breathing (equal counts for inhale, hold, exhale, and hold) to reduce anxiety.

36. Practice progressive muscle relaxation by inhaling deeply and tensing muscles, then exhaling while releasing tension.

37. Use your breath to enhance the effects of stretching and relaxation exercises.

Posture Correction:

38. Set reminders to check your posture throughout the day and adjust as needed.

39. Use a lumbar support cushion when sitting for prolonged periods to maintain proper spinal alignment.

40. Keep your computer monitor at eye level to prevent slouching and neck strain.

41. Use ergonomic chairs and keyboards to support proper posture during work.

42. Perform regular posture check-ins during your daily routine.

Tips for Integrating Physical Manipulation:

43. Start your morning with a brief stretching routine to wake up your body.

44. Incorporate a few minutes of deep breathing exercises into your daily mindfulness practice.

45. Set a timer to remind yourself to stand up, stretch, and adjust your posture throughout the day.

46. Create a dedicated space for stretching and relaxation exercises in your home.

47. Use guided meditation apps that incorporate gentle movement and physical manipulation.

Holistic Wellness:

48. Combine physical manipulation with aromatherapy for a sensory-enhanced relaxation experience.

49. Practice physical manipulation techniques before bedtime to promote relaxation and better sleep.

50. Combine stretching with breathing exercises for a calming and invigorating routine.

51. Incorporate physical manipulation into your self-care routine to reduce stress and enhance well-being.

52. Use manipulation techniques as part of your warm-up and cooldown routine during exercise.

Relaxation and Stress Reduction:

53. Perform a full-body stretch routine before bedtime to unwind and relax your muscles.

54. Use self-massage techniques on your hands and wrists after typing for extended periods.

55. Try deep breathing exercises during stressful moments to regain a sense of calm.

56. Create a calming atmosphere with soft lighting, soothing music, and aromatherapy.

57. Incorporate manipulation techniques into your relaxation routine to fully release tension.

Targeted Relief:

58. If you have tension headaches, focus on acupressure points on the head and neck.

59. If you experience lower back discomfort, practice stretches that target the lower back and hip muscles.

60. For tight hamstrings, incorporate gentle stretches and self-myofascial release techniques.

61. If you have tight shoulders, perform shoulder rolls and massage to release tension.

62. Address stiffness in your hands and wrists with gentle stretching and self-massage.

Complementing Other Remedies:

63. Use physical manipulation alongside hot/cold therapy to alleviate muscle discomfort.

64. Combine stretching with herbal remedies to support overall muscle health.

65. Pair physical manipulation with relaxation techniques for enhanced stress relief.

66. Use manipulation techniques to enhance the effects of aromatherapy during relaxation sessions.

67. Combine acupressure with breathing exercises to alleviate tension and promote relaxation.

Mindful Movement:

68. Practice mindfulness while performing manipulation techniques to fully experience the benefits.

69. Incorporate physical manipulation into your yoga or meditation practice for a holistic experience.

70. Use movement and manipulation to connect with your body and promote self-awareness.

Creating a Routine:

71. Design a daily routine that includes a few minutes of stretching and manipulation.

72. Use weekends as an opportunity for more extended stretching and relaxation sessions.

73. Create a visual schedule or checklist to track your manipulation practices.

74. Share your routines with friends or family members to encourage accountability.

Safe Practice:

75. Listen to your body and never push yourself beyond your comfort zone.

76. If you have existing health conditions or injuries, consult a healthcare professional before trying new manipulation techniques.

77. Start with gentle movements and progress gradually as your body becomes more accustomed.

78. Stay hydrated before and after practicing manipulation to support muscle health.

Variety and Exploration:

79. Explore different types of manipulation techniques to find what works best for you.

80. Rotate through various stretching routines to target different muscle groups.

81. Experiment with self-massage tools like massage balls, foam rollers, and massage sticks.

82. Try different breathing exercises to find the ones that resonate with you.

Incorporate Into Daily Activities:

83. Practice stretching and manipulation while watching TV or listening to a podcast.

84. Use manipulation techniques during breaks at work or study sessions to relieve tension.

85. Incorporate deep breathing into your morning routine to start your day with calm and focus.

86. Combine stretching and manipulation with mindfulness during daily walks.

Mind-Body Connection:

87. Practice physical manipulation with an intention in mind, such as stress relief or improved flexibility.

88. Use manipulation techniques as an opportunity to practice mindfulness and connect with your body.

Family and Social:

89. Encourage your family members to join you in stretching and manipulation routines.

90. Share your favorite techniques with friends and create a support network for well-being practices.

91. Incorporate physical manipulation into family bonding time or gatherings.

Explore Online Resources:

92. Access online videos and tutorials for guided stretching and manipulation sessions.

93. Join online forums or communities to learn from others' experiences and share your own.

94. Follow reputable wellness influencers or practitioners who offer insights into manipulation techniques.

Consistency and Long-Term Benefits:

95. Embrace a long-term perspective on physical manipulation, focusing on gradual improvement.

96. Celebrate small milestones, such as increased flexibility or reduced discomfort.

97. Remember that regular practice yields cumulative benefits for physical and mental well-being.

Tailored to Your Needs:

98. Customize your manipulation routines to address your specific discomforts and goals.

99. Modify techniques based on your body's feedback and any changes you notice over time.

100. Embrace physical manipulation as a personalized, ongoing practice that supports your overall health and wellness.

Remember that the effectiveness of physical manipulation varies for each individual, and it's important to listen to your body and practice techniques that feel comfortable and safe. If you have any underlying health conditions or concerns, consult a healthcare professional before incorporating new manipulation practices into your routine.

Homeopathic remedies

Homeopathic remedies are a type of alternative medicine that involves using highly diluted substances derived from natural sources to stimulate the body's innate healing abilities. Homeopathy is based on the principle of "like cures like," meaning that a substance that can cause symptoms in a healthy person can be used in a highly diluted form to treat similar symptoms in an individual with an illness.

Homeopathic remedies are believed to work on an energetic level, aiming to restore balance and promote self-healing. Here's a deeper look into homeopathic remedies as a type of home remedy:

Principles of Homeopathy:

1. **Similars:** The foundation of homeopathy is the principle of treating "like with like." This means that a substance that produces certain symptoms in a healthy person can be used to treat similar symptoms in a sick person.

2. **Minimum Dose:** Homeopathic remedies are highly diluted, often to the point where the original substance is virtually undetectable. It's believed that the energetic imprint of the substance remains and stimulates the body's healing response.

3. **Holistic Approach:** Homeopathy considers the person as a whole, taking into account physical, mental, and emotional aspects. Treatment is tailored to the individual's unique symptoms and constitution.

4. **Vital Force:** Homeopathy focuses on the body's vital force or life energy. Imbalances in this vital force are believed to manifest as symptoms of illness.

How Homeopathic Remedies Are Prepared:

1. **Serial Dilution:** The process involves diluting the original substance in water or alcohol and then vigorously shaking or succussing the mixture. This process is repeated multiple times, resulting in high dilutions.

2. **Potentization:** Dilutions are given potency levels, denoted by numbers such as 6X, 30C, etc. The higher the potency, the more diluted and potent the remedy is believed to be.

3. **Infinitesimal Concentrations:** In many cases, the final homeopathic remedy may not contain a single molecule of the original substance. Instead, it carries the energetic imprint.

Common Uses of Homeopathic Remedies:

1. **Acute Ailments:** Homeopathic remedies are often used to address acute conditions like colds, flu, headaches, and minor injuries.

2. **Chronic Conditions:** Some people turn to homeopathy for chronic conditions such as allergies, digestive issues, skin problems, and emotional imbalances.

3. **Behavioral Issues:** Homeopathic remedies are also used to address certain behavioral issues, anxiety, and sleep disturbances.

4. **Women's Health:** Homeopathy is sometimes used to address menstrual irregularities, menopausal symptoms, and pregnancy-related discomfort.

Safety and Considerations:

1. **Individualized Approach:** Homeopathic remedies are selected based on the person's unique symptoms and constitution. What works for one person may not work for another.

2. **Professional Consultation:** It's advisable to consult a trained and licensed homeopath to receive appropriate remedies and dosages tailored to your needs.

3. **Holistic Assessment:** A homeopath considers your physical, emotional, and mental state to determine the appropriate remedy.

4. **Complementary Approach:** Homeopathic remedies can be used alongside conventional medical treatments as a complementary approach.

5. **Placebo Effect:** Some studies suggest that the benefits of homeopathy might be attributed to the placebo effect. It's essential to approach homeopathy with an open but critical mind.

Tips for Using Homeopathic Remedies:

1. **Consult a Professional:** Seek guidance from a qualified homeopath who can assess your symptoms and recommend appropriate remedies.

2. **Follow Recommendations:** Take the prescribed remedy as directed by the homeopath. The timing and frequency matter.

3. **Avoid Strong Flavors:** Avoid consuming strong flavors (mint, coffee, etc.) around the time of taking homeopathic remedies.

4. **Storage:** Store remedies away from strong odors, heat, and direct sunlight.

5. **Individualized Approach:** Different people with the same condition might receive different remedies based on their unique symptoms.

6. **Keep Records:** Maintain a journal of symptoms and responses to homeopathic remedies to track progress.

Homeopathic remedies are a distinctive type of alternative medicine that operates on the principle of using highly diluted substances to stimulate the body's healing response. While it's a practice with a long history, its effectiveness and mechanisms of action remain a subject of debate. If you're considering homeopathy, it's advisable to seek guidance from a qualified homeopath and approach it with an open but informed perspective.

100 tips for using homeopathic remedies effectively as a type of home remedy:

Choosing and Using Homeopathic Remedies:

1. **Consult a Professional:** Seek guidance from a qualified homeopath for accurate remedy selection based on your individual symptoms and constitution.

2. **Educate Yourself:** Learn about the basic principles of homeopathy to understand how remedies work.

3. **Research Trusted Sources:** Explore reputable books, websites, and resources to gain insights into different remedies.

4. **Dosage and Potency:** Follow the recommended dosage and potency as prescribed by the homeopath.

5. **Keep Records:** Maintain a symptom journal to track changes and responses to different remedies.

6. **Single Remedies:** Start with single remedies rather than complex combinations for better assessment.

7. **Avoid Self-Diagnosis:** Do not self-diagnose; rely on a professional homeopath's assessment for accurate remedy selection.

8. **Store Properly:** Keep remedies away from strong odors, heat, sunlight, and electromagnetic fields.

9. **Avoid Strong Tastes:** Refrain from consuming strong-tasting substances (coffee, mint, etc.) around the time of taking remedies.

10. **Consistency Matters:** Stick to the recommended dosing schedule consistently for optimal results.

Safety and Compatibility:

11. **Inform Your Healthcare Provider:** Inform your conventional healthcare provider about any homeopathic remedies you're taking.

12. **Allergies and Sensitivities:** Mention any allergies or sensitivities to your homeopath to avoid remedies with potential triggers.

13. **Children and Pregnancy:** Consult a professional before administering remedies to children, pregnant individuals, or nursing mothers.

14. **Drug Interactions:** Discuss possible interactions with conventional medications or supplements with your homeopath.

15. **Follow Professional Guidance:** Adhere to the recommendations of your homeopath for remedy selection and dosing.

Managing Acute Conditions:

16. **Flu and Colds:** Homeopathic remedies like Oscillococcinum can be used at the onset of flu symptoms.

17. **Headaches:** Choose a remedy based on the type of headache (e.g., Belladonna for sudden, throbbing headaches).

18. **Indigestion:** Consider remedies like Nux Vomica for overindulgence or Carbo Veg for bloating.

19. **Injuries:** Arnica montana is a commonly used remedy for minor injuries and bruises.

20. **Allergies:** Seek remedies like Allium Cepa for hay fever symptoms or Histaminum for allergy relief.

21. **Insomnia:** Choose remedies like Coffea Cruda for racing thoughts or Ignatia for sleeplessness due to grief.

22. **Nausea:** Remedies like Ipecacuanha or Nux Vomica can help with different types of nausea.

Chronic Conditions:

23. **Eczema:** Consider remedies like Sulphur or Graphites based on individual symptoms and triggers.

24. **Anxiety:** Remedies like Aconite, Gelsemium, or Argentum Nitricum may be used for different anxiety presentations.

25. **Arthritis:** Remedies like Rhus Toxicodendron or Bryonia may help with joint pain and stiffness.

26. **Asthma:** Consult a professional for remedies like Arsenicum Album or Natrum Sulphuricum for asthma symptoms.

27. **Menstrual Issues:** Remedies like Pulsatilla or Sepia can be considered for menstrual irregularities.

28. **Depression:** Consult a professional for appropriate remedies based on individual emotional and mental states.

Preventive Care:

29. **Travel Ailments:** Use remedies like Cocculus Indicus for motion sickness or Jet Lag formulas for travel fatigue.

30. **Immune Support:** Consider homeopathic immune boosters like Echinacea or influenzinum for seasonal protection.

31. **Cold Prevention:** Choose remedies like Eupatorium Perfoliatum or Ferrum Phosphoricum at the onset of cold symptoms.

32. **Stress Management:** Remedies like Ignatia or Lycopodium can be considered for stress and emotional well-being.

Mind-Body Connection:

33. **Meditation and Remedies:** Combine meditation practices with remedies to support emotional balance.

34. **Mindful Consumption:** Engage in mindful eating and lifestyle choices to complement the effects of homeopathic remedies.

35. **Positive Affirmations:** Incorporate positive affirmations alongside remedies to support overall well-being.

Holistic Approach:

36. **Holistic Assessment:** Consider physical, mental, and emotional symptoms to select remedies that address the whole person.

37. **Individualized Treatment:** Tailor remedy choices to your unique constitution, preferences, and health history.

38. **Lifestyle Modifications:** Make supportive lifestyle changes to complement the effects of homeopathic remedies.

Safe Practice:

39. **Professional Consultation:** Always consult a professional for complex or chronic conditions to receive appropriate remedies.

40. **Avoid Overdosing:** Stick to the recommended dosages and avoid overusing remedies.

41. **Monitor Reactions:** Keep track of your body's responses to remedies and adjust if needed.

42. **Know When to Stop:** If symptoms worsen or new symptoms arise, consult a professional.

Supplementing with Nutrients:

43. **Nutritional Support:** Combine homeopathic remedies with nutritional supplements to enhance overall health.

44. **Vitamin and Mineral Balance:** Consider using homeopathic remedies to support deficiencies in conjunction with dietary changes.

Mindfulness and Relaxation:

45. **Mind-Body Practices:** Integrate practices like yoga, meditation, and deep breathing alongside homeopathic remedies.

46. **Holistic Wellness:** Combine relaxation techniques with remedies for a comprehensive approach to well-being.

Combining with Other Remedies:

47. **Hot/Cold Therapy:** Use homeopathic remedies alongside hot or cold therapy for muscle relief.

48. **Aromatherapy:** Combine aromatherapy with remedies for an enhanced sensory experience.

Creating a Healing Space:

49. **Aromatherapy Diffusion:** Use diffused essential oils in your healing space while taking homeopathic remedies.

50. **Comfortable Environment:** Create a calm and comfortable environment to support healing while taking remedies.

Mental and Emotional Health:

51. **Journaling:** Maintain a journal to track emotional changes and responses to homeopathic remedies.

52. **Mindfulness Meditation:** Practice mindfulness meditation alongside remedies for emotional balance.

Physical Activity and Movement:

53. **Stretching and Exercise:** Combine regular stretching or exercise with homeopathic remedies for overall well-being.

54. **Yoga Practice:** Integrate yoga poses and breathing techniques to enhance the effects of remedies.

Exploring Personal Growth:

55. **Self-Reflection:** Engage in self-reflection practices to understand how remedies impact your well-being.

56. **Visualization:** Practice visualization techniques alongside remedies for holistic healing.

Balancing Energy:

57. **Energy Healing:** Explore energy healing modalities like Reiki or acupuncture alongside homeopathic remedies.

Sharing Experiences:

58. **Supportive Community:** Connect with others who use homeopathic remedies for shared experiences and insights.

59. **Sharing Tips:** Exchange tips and remedies with friends or online communities to broaden your knowledge.

Mindful Nutrition:

60. **Whole Foods:** Choose whole, nutrient-dense foods to support overall health while using homeopathic remedies.

61. **Herbal Teas:** Pair homeopathic remedies with herbal teas for a soothing and supportive approach.

Intuitive Healing:

62. **Trust Your Intuition:** Tune into your body's responses to remedies and adjust based on your intuition.

Positive Lifestyle Choices:

63. **Positive Affirmations:** Pair positive affirmations with remedies to support a positive mindset.

64. **Healthy Sleep Habits:** Prioritize sleep hygiene practices alongside homeopathic remedies for better sleep.

Mindful Breathing:

65. **Breathing Exercises:** Practice mindful breathing exercises to enhance the effects of homeopathic remedies.

Holistic Nurturing:

66. **Nature Connection:** Spend time in nature to complement the holistic effects of homeopathic remedies.

67. **Mindful Walks:** Take mindful walks outdoors while reflecting on the healing process.

Creative Expression:

68. **Art and Creativity:** Engage in artistic or creative activities alongside homeopathic remedies for holistic nurturing.

69. **Journaling:** Write down thoughts, emotions, and responses to remedies as a form of creative expression.

Spiritual Connection:

70. **Meditative Practices:** Incorporate meditation and mindfulness practices for a deeper spiritual connection while using remedies.

71. **Prayer or Affirmations:** Pair spiritual practices with homeopathic remedies for a holistic approach.

Breathing and Relaxation:

72. **Relaxation Techniques:** Practice relaxation exercises like progressive muscle relaxation alongside remedies.

Supportive Relationships:

73. **Caring Connections:** Share your homeopathic journey with loved ones for supportive relationships.

Holistic Well-Being:

74. **Integrated Approach:** Use homeopathic remedies in conjunction with other holistic approaches to well-being.

75. **Self-Care Rituals:** Create self-care rituals that include homeopathic remedies for daily nurturing.

Individualized Approaches:

76. **Tailor Remedies:** Choose remedies that resonate with your individual physical, mental, and emotional state.

Mindful Eating:

77. **Mindful Meals:** Practice mindful eating alongside remedies to enhance their effects on well-being.

78. **Nutrient-Rich Diet:** Consume nutrient-rich foods that complement the effects of homeopathic remedies.

Emotional Healing:

79. **Emotional Release:** Pair homeopathic remedies with emotional release techniques for holistic healing.

Positive Mindset:

80. **Gratitude Practice:** Cultivate a gratitude practice to support a positive mindset while using remedies.

81. **Visualization:** Visualize wellness and healing while taking homeopathic remedies.

Holistic Healing:

82. **Body-Mind Connection:** Recognize the interconnectedness of the body and mind while using remedies.

Awareness and Presence:

83. **Present-Moment Awareness:** Practice being present in the moment while using homeopathic remedies.

84. **Breathing Meditation:** Pair remedies with breathing meditation for mindful healing.

Holistic Rituals:

85. **Rituals of Self-Care:** Incorporate homeopathic remedies into self-care rituals for holistic nurturing.

Energy Balancing:

86. **Energy Practices:** Explore energy-balancing practices like Qigong or Tai Chi alongside homeopathic remedies.

Holistic Connection:

87. **Holistic Practitioner:** Consult holistic practitioners who combine homeopathy with other modalities.

Personal Evolution:

88. **Personal Growth:** Use homeopathic remedies to support your personal growth and evolution.

Physical Connection:

89. **Physical Touch:** Incorporate physical touch and comforting gestures while using homeopathic remedies.

Holistic Awareness:

90. **Body Scan:** Practice a body scan meditation while taking remedies to enhance awareness.

Holistic Healing Environment:

91. **Sacred Space:** Create a sacred space for taking remedies to enhance their holistic effects.

Holistic Nurturing:

92. **Caring for Self:** Nourish your physical, emotional, and mental well-being while using remedies.

Nature's Healing:

93. **Nature's Remedies:** Explore nature's healing remedies alongside homeopathic approaches.

Exploration and Curiosity:

94. **Open-Mindedness:** Approach homeopathy with curiosity and an open mind.

Balancing Energies:

95. **Chakra Balancing:** Explore chakra balancing practices alongside homeopathic remedies.

Holistic Nutrition:

96. **Balanced Diet:** Support remedies with a balanced diet that nourishes your entire being.

Mindful Lifestyle:

97. **Mindful Choices:** Make conscious lifestyle choices that align with your holistic well-being.

Positive Intentions:

98. **Intentions for Healing:** Set positive intentions for healing while using homeopathic remedies.

Wholeness and Balance:

99. **Wholeness Within:** Recognize the importance of holistic balance within the body and mind.

100. **Holistic Wellness:** Embrace homeopathic remedies as part of your journey towards holistic wellness.

Remember that while homeopathic remedies have been used by many individuals, their effectiveness varies from person to person. It's important to approach homeopathy with an open but informed perspective and to seek guidance from qualified professionals for optimal results.

Mind-body practices

Mind-body practices, also known as mind-body medicine or mind-body therapies, are a type of home remedy that focuses on the interconnectedness of the mind, emotions, and body to promote overall health and well-being. These practices recognize the powerful influence of psychological and emotional factors on physical health. The goal of mind-body practices is to create harmony between the mind and body, enhancing the body's natural healing mechanisms. Here's a deeper exploration of mind-body practices as a type of home remedy:

Principles of Mind-Body Practices:

1. **Holistic Perspective:** Mind-body practices consider the body and mind as interconnected aspects of health, influencing each other in complex ways.

2. **Self-Healing:** These practices aim to activate the body's innate healing capacities by addressing mental, emotional, and physical aspects simultaneously.

3. **Stress Reduction:** Mind-body practices often emphasize stress reduction as chronic stress can negatively impact physical health.

4. **Mindfulness and Awareness:** Many mind-body techniques encourage being present in the moment, fostering self-awareness and consciousness.

Common Mind-Body Practices:

1. **Meditation:** Meditation involves focusing the mind to achieve a heightened state of awareness, relaxation, and tranquility. Various forms of meditation exist, including mindfulness, loving-kindness, and transcendental meditation.

2. **Yoga:** Yoga combines physical postures, breathing exercises, and meditation to promote flexibility, balance, and relaxation. It addresses both physical fitness and mental calmness.

3. **Tai Chi:** Tai Chi is a Chinese martial art that involves slow, flowing movements and deep breathing. It promotes balance, flexibility, and relaxation.

4. **Qi Gong:** Qi Gong is a Chinese practice that combines gentle movements, breathing, and meditation to enhance the body's vital energy (qi) flow.

5. **Breathwork:** Conscious breathing techniques focus on controlling the breath to promote relaxation, reduce stress, and increase mindfulness.

6. **Progressive Muscle Relaxation:** This technique involves tensing and relaxing different muscle groups to promote relaxation and reduce muscle tension.

7. **Guided Imagery:** Guided imagery uses mental visualization to create calming and positive mental images, fostering relaxation and reducing stress.

8. **Biofeedback:** Biofeedback uses electronic monitoring to provide real-time information about physiological functions like heart rate or muscle tension, enabling individuals to learn to control these functions.

9. **Autogenic Training:** This technique involves repeating specific phrases to induce a state of relaxation and self-suggestion.

10. **Hypnotherapy:** Hypnotherapy uses guided relaxation and focused attention to achieve a heightened state of awareness, enabling changes in thoughts, feelings, and behaviors.

Benefits of Mind-Body Practices:

- **Stress Reduction:** Mind-body practices help manage stress and promote relaxation, leading to reduced stress-related health issues.

- **Emotional Well-being:** These practices enhance emotional resilience, reduce anxiety, and promote a positive outlook on life.

- **Physical Health:** Mind-body practices have been associated with improved cardiovascular health, immune function, and pain management.

- **Mindfulness:** Practicing mindfulness increases present-moment awareness and cultivates a nonjudgmental attitude towards thoughts and feelings.

- **Psychological Benefits:** Mind-body practices support better sleep, enhanced focus, and reduced symptoms of depression.

- **Holistic Balance:** These practices encourage harmony between mental, emotional, and physical aspects of health.

Incorporating Mind-Body Practices:

1. **Consistency:** Dedicate regular time for mind-body practices, whether daily or a few times a week, to experience their benefits.

2. **Start Small:** Begin with short sessions and gradually increase the duration as you become more comfortable.

3. **Personalize:** Explore different practices to find what resonates with you and meets your needs.

4. **Create a Calm Space:** Practice in a quiet, comfortable space that supports relaxation and focus.

5. **Breathing Awareness:** Begin many mind-body practices with focusing on your breath, which anchors you in the present moment.

6. **Mindful Eating:** Practice mindful eating by savoring each bite, paying attention to flavors, textures, and sensations.

7. **Self-Compassion:** Approach these practices with self-compassion and non-judgment, letting go of expectations.

8. **Supportive Community:** Join mindfulness groups or classes to connect with others and enhance your practice.

Mind-Body Practices and Specific Conditions:

- **Stress:** Mind-body practices are particularly effective in managing stress and its related physical and emotional effects.

- **Anxiety and Depression:** These practices can alleviate symptoms and support emotional well-being.

- **Chronic Pain:** Mind-body practices like yoga and meditation can complement pain management strategies.

- **Cardiovascular Health:** Practices like meditation and tai chi may contribute to better heart health.

- **Sleep Disorders:** Mind-body practices improve sleep quality and address insomnia.

Complementary and Integrative Approach:

- **Holistic Wellness:** Combine mind-body practices with other home remedies like herbal remedies, aromatherapy, and dietary changes.

- **Professional Guidance:** If you have specific health concerns, consult healthcare professionals before incorporating mind-body practices into your routine.

Mind-body practices are a valuable type of home remedy that promotes the integration of mental, emotional, and physical well-being. By fostering relaxation, reducing stress, and enhancing self-awareness, these practices support overall health and create a harmonious balance between mind and body. Incorporating mind-body practices into your daily routine can contribute to holistic well-being and resilience in the face of life's challenges.

100 tips for effectively using mind-body practices as a type of home remedy for holistic well-being:

General Tips:

1. **Start Slowly:** Begin with short sessions and gradually extend your practice as you become more comfortable.

2. **Consistency Matters:** Establish a regular routine for mind-body practices to experience lasting benefits.

3. **Mindful Beginnings:** Start your day with a brief mindfulness session to set a positive tone.

4. **Before Sleep:** Wind down with relaxation techniques before bedtime for better sleep quality.

5. **Choose Your Practice:** Explore different mind-body practices to find the one that resonates with you.

6. **Create a Sacred Space:** Set up a dedicated, clutter-free space for your practice to enhance focus.

7. **Comfort is Key:** Use cushions, blankets, and comfortable clothing to ensure physical comfort.

8. **Silence or Music:** Choose a quiet environment or play soothing music to enhance relaxation.

9. **Tech-Free Zone:** Keep electronic devices away during your practice to minimize distractions.

10. **Open-Mindedness:** Approach practices with an open mind, allowing yourself to explore and learn.

11. **Set Intentions:** Begin each practice with a positive intention or affirmation.

12. **Breathing Awareness:** Start with breath awareness to anchor your mind in the present moment.

13. **Release Expectations:** Let go of perfectionism; every practice is a learning experience.

14. **Be Patient:** Results may take time; trust the process and be patient with yourself.

15. **Journaling:** Keep a practice journal to track your experiences, insights, and progress.

16. **Personalize:** Modify practices to suit your preferences and adapt as needed.

17. **Mix and Match:** Combine different practices for a comprehensive mind-body experience.

18. **Self-Care Priority:** Prioritize self-care and dedicate time to your practice regularly.

19. **Practice Gratitude:** Incorporate moments of gratitude into your practice to cultivate positivity.

20. **Stay Present:** Gently bring your focus back whenever your mind wanders during practice.

21. **Breath Breaks:** Take short mindful breathing breaks throughout the day to refresh your mind.

22. **Visualization:** Incorporate guided visualizations to enhance relaxation and positive thinking.

23. **Walking Meditation:** Practice mindfulness while walking, focusing on each step and your breath.

24. **Progressive Relaxation:** Use progressive muscle relaxation to release physical tension.

25. **Mindful Chores:** Engage mindfully in daily chores, using them as opportunities for practice.

Meditation:

26. **Morning Meditation:** Start your day with a guided meditation to set a peaceful tone.

27. **Mindful Eating:** Eat one meal mindfully, savoring each bite and engaging all your senses.

28. **Body Scan:** Practice a body scan meditation to cultivate body awareness and relaxation.

29. **Loving-Kindness:** Practice loving-kindness meditation to cultivate compassion for yourself and others.

30. **Breath Meditation:** Focus on your breath, observing its natural rhythm and sensations.

31. **Nature Meditation:** Meditate outdoors, connecting with nature's sights and sounds.

32. **Gratitude Meditation:** Reflect on moments of gratitude during your meditation practice.

33. **Creative Meditation:** Engage in creative activities like drawing or writing after meditation.

34. **Guided Meditation Apps:** Explore guided meditation apps for a variety of practices and themes.

Yoga:

35. **Morning Yoga:** Start your day with a gentle yoga flow to awaken your body and mind.

36. **Stretch Breaks:** Take short yoga breaks during the day to release tension and increase flexibility.

37. **Sun Salutations:** Practice sun salutations to invigorate your body and mind.

38. **Restorative Yoga:** Wind down with restorative poses and deep breathing before sleep.

39. **Partner Yoga:** Practice yoga with a partner or family member for a shared experience.

40. **Online Classes:** Explore online yoga classes for guided sessions tailored to your level.

41. **Yoga Nidra:** Experience deep relaxation with yoga nidra sessions for mental clarity.

42. **Mindful Transitions:** Practice mindful movement during transitions between poses.

Tai Chi and Qi Gong:

43. **Tai Chi Flow:** Follow a tai chi routine to promote balance, flexibility, and tranquility.

44. **Qi Gong Energy:** Practice qi gong exercises to balance your body's energy flow.

45. **Breathing with Movements:** Coordinate your breath with tai chi or qi gong movements.

Breathwork:

46. **Diaphragmatic Breathing:** Practice diaphragmatic breathing to activate the body's relaxation response.

47. **4-7-8 Technique:** Inhale for 4 counts, hold for 7 counts, exhale for 8 counts to promote calmness.

48. **Alternate Nostril Breathing:** Use this technique to balance energy and calm the mind.

49. **Box Breathing:** Inhale, hold, exhale, and hold for equal counts in a square pattern.

Guided Imagery and Visualization:

50. **Healing Imagery:** Imagine healing light or energy flowing through your body, promoting wellness.

51. **Nature Visualization:** Visualize yourself in a peaceful natural setting to promote relaxation.

52. **Dreamscape Visualization:** Create your dream world during visualization practice.

Biofeedback:

53. **Heart Rate Variability:** Use apps or devices to monitor heart rate variability and practice coherence breathing.

54. **Muscle Tension Feedback:** Use biofeedback devices to identify and release muscle tension.

Autogenic Training and Hypnotherapy:

55. **Autogenic Phrases:** Repeat autogenic phrases like "I am calm and relaxed" for relaxation.

56. **Positive Affirmations:** Integrate positive affirmations during autogenic training or hypnotherapy.

Mind-Body Integration:

57. **Mindful Movement:** Practice mindful walking, paying attention to each step and your breath.

58. **Body-Mind Connection:** Notice how emotions and thoughts manifest in your body during practice.

59. **Breath Awareness:** Observe how your breath changes with different emotions or thoughts.

Integration with Daily Activities:

60. **Mindful Eating:** Engage in mindful eating during meals, savoring each bite.

61. **Mindful Showering:** Focus on the sensations of water and cleansing while showering.

62. **Mindful Driving:** Pay full attention while driving, engaging all your senses.

Holistic Well-Being:

63. **Self-Compassion:** Practice self-compassion during mind-body practices, cultivating kindness towards yourself.

64. **Stress Relief:** Use mind-body practices to release stress and promote relaxation.

65. **Emotional Balance:** Practice to regulate emotions and maintain emotional well-being.

66. **Physical Alignment:** Focus on alignment and posture during mind-body practices to support physical health.

67. **Holistic Healing:** View mind-body practices as part of your holistic healing journey.

Mindful Communication:

68. **Listening Mindfully:** Practice active listening during conversations, fully present without judgment.

69. **Mindful Speech:** Speak mindfully, choosing words consciously and with intention.

Mind-Body Integration Techniques:

70. **Breath and Movement:** Sync your breath with movement to enhance mind-body connection.

71. **Focused Attention:** Direct your attention to a specific body part to enhance awareness.

72. **Progressive Relaxation:** Tense and release muscle groups, promoting physical and mental relaxation.

Mindful Lifestyle Choices:

73. **Mindful Technology Use:** Use electronic devices mindfully, setting intentional usage times.

74. **Mindful Eating:** Consume whole foods mindfully, paying attention to taste and texture.

75. **Mindful Activities:** Engage in activities with full presence, immersing yourself in the experience.

Holistic Time Management:

76. **Time for Reflection:** Allocate time for self-reflection and mindfulness throughout the day.

77. **Scheduled Practice:** Include scheduled mind-body breaks in your daily routine.

Mindful Stress Management:

78. **Stress Check-ins:** Pause periodically to check in with your stress levels and practice relaxation.

79. **Breath Breaks:** Take deep breaths whenever stress arises, diffusing tension.

80. **Mindful Breaks:** Take short mindful breaks during work to rejuvenate your mind.

Emotional Regulation:

81. **Emotional Release:** Allow yourself to express and release emotions during practice.

82. **Emotion Observance:** Notice how different emotions manifest in your body during practice.

Gratitude and Positivity:

83. **Gratitude Journal:** Maintain a journal to note down moments of gratitude during practice.

84. **Positive Affirmations:** Integrate positive affirmations into your practice for a positive mindset.

Mindful Sleep Preparation:

85. **Bedtime Relaxation:** Engage in a relaxation practice before sleep to prepare your mind and body.

86. **Sleep Visualization:** Visualize a peaceful sleep scene to enhance relaxation and sleep quality.

Holistic Self-Care:

87. **Mindful Bathing:** Take mindful baths, focusing on the sensations of water and relaxation.

88. **Mindful Grooming:** Engage in grooming routines with full attention and presence.

Mind-Body Awareness:

89. **Bodily Sensations:** Notice physical sensations during practice, fostering body awareness.

90. **Thought Observation:** Observe passing thoughts without judgment, letting them come and go.

Mindful Relationships:

91. **Listening Mindfully:** Practice active listening in relationships, focusing fully on the speaker.

92. **Mindful Conversations:** Engage in conversations with full presence and genuine interest.

Mindful Parenting:

93. **Parent-Child Bonding:** Engage in mindful interactions with your children, being fully present.

94. **Modeling Mindfulness:** Demonstrate mindfulness practices to children through your actions.

Mindful Nature Connection:

95. **Outdoor Mindfulness:** Practice mindfulness outdoors, connecting with nature's beauty.

96. **Nature Meditation:** Meditate in a natural setting, absorbing its tranquility and energy.

Self-Compassion and Forgiveness:

97. **Self-Forgiveness:** Practice self-forgiveness during mind-body practices, letting go of self-criticism.

98. **Self-Kindness:** Be kind to yourself during practice, cultivating self-compassion.

Mindful Creativity:

99. **Creative Expression:** Engage in creative activities mindfully, immersing yourself in the creative process.

100. **Creative Visualization:** Visualize creative projects coming to fruition during mindfulness practice.

Remember that mind-body practices are a personal journey, and these tips can be adapted to suit your individual needs and preferences. Experiment with different approaches to find what resonates with you and enhances your well-being.

DIY beauty and skincare

DIY beauty and skincare are types of home remedies that involve creating your own natural and holistic beauty products using readily available ingredients. These remedies emphasize using natural, non-toxic ingredients to nourish and enhance your skin and hair. DIY beauty and skincare methods allow you to have more control over what you apply to your body, and they often come with the added benefits of cost-effectiveness and customization. Here's a deeper look into DIY beauty and skincare as a type of home remedy:

Benefits of DIY Beauty and Skincare:

1. **Natural Ingredients:** DIY beauty recipes often utilize natural ingredients like fruits, herbs, oils, and essential oils, minimizing exposure to harmful chemicals.

2. **Customization:** You can tailor DIY products to your skin type, concerns, and preferences, creating a personalized skincare routine.

3. **Cost-Effectiveness:** Making your own products can be more affordable in the long run compared to store-bought options.

4. **Creativity:** DIY beauty allows you to experiment with various ingredients and formulations.

5. **Environmental Impact:** Using natural and homemade products can be more environmentally friendly by reducing packaging waste and chemical runoff.

Common DIY Beauty and Skincare Products:

1. **Cleansers:** Homemade cleansers often include gentle ingredients like honey, yogurt, oatmeal, or aloe vera gel.

2. **Facial Scrubs:** Exfoliate with natural ingredients like sugar, salt, coffee grounds, or ground oats.

3. **Face Masks:** Create masks with ingredients such as clay, avocado, banana, turmeric, or yogurt.

4. **Toners:** Use witch hazel, rose water, green tea, or apple cider vinegar as toners.

5. **Serums:** DIY serums might include vitamin C, hyaluronic acid, and nourishing oils.

6. **Moisturizers:** Make moisturizers using shea butter, coconut oil, jojoba oil, or aloe vera.

7. **Lip Balms:** Mix beeswax, coconut oil, and essential oils for natural lip care.

8. **Hair Masks:** Nourish your hair with homemade masks containing coconut oil, yogurt, honey, and eggs.

9. **Body Scrubs:** Create exfoliating body scrubs with salt or sugar and moisturizing oils.

10. **Body Lotions:** Blend shea butter, cocoa butter, and essential oils for luxurious body lotions.

DIY Beauty and Skincare Tips:

1. **Patch Test:** Always do a patch test before using a new DIY product to ensure you're not allergic or sensitive to any ingredient.

2. **Fresh Ingredients:** Use fresh and organic ingredients whenever possible for optimal results.

3. **Clean Tools:** Ensure your hands, utensils, and containers are clean before creating DIY products.

4. **Storage:** Store homemade products in a cool, dark place to prevent spoilage.

5. **Labeling:** Label your creations with the date and ingredients to track their freshness.

6. **Expiration Dates:** Many DIY products have shorter shelf lives due to the absence of preservatives, so use them within a reasonable time frame.

7. **Consistency:** Consistent use of DIY products is important to see noticeable results over time.

8. **Hygiene:** Avoid dipping fingers directly into jars to prevent contamination; use clean spatulas or droppers.

9. **Gentle Ingredients:** Opt for gentle ingredients, especially if you have sensitive or reactive skin.

10. **Sun Protection:** If your DIY products will be used during the day, consider adding natural sun protection like zinc oxide or red raspberry seed oil.

11. **Simple Formulas:** Start with simple DIY recipes and gradually experiment with more complex formulations.

12. **Research:** Research the properties of ingredients before using them to ensure they suit your needs.

13. **Avoid Irritants:** Avoid ingredients that are known allergens or skin irritants.

14. **Consultation:** If you have serious skin concerns or conditions, consult a dermatologist before using DIY products.

15. **Take Notes:** Keep a journal of your DIY beauty experiments, noting what works best for your skin.

16. **Remove Makeup:** Always remove makeup and cleanse your face before applying any DIY product.

17. **Moderation:** Don't overuse DIY treatments; excessive exfoliation or use of potent ingredients can lead to irritation.

18. **Be Patient:** Natural remedies often take time to show results, so be patient and consistent.

DIY Beauty and Skincare Ingredient Ideas:

1. **Honey:** Moisturizes, soothes, and has antibacterial properties.

2. **Coconut Oil:** Nourishes and hydrates skin and hair.

3. **Aloe Vera Gel:** Calms irritation and hydrates.

4. **Oats:** Soothes and gently exfoliates.

5. **Green Tea:** Contains antioxidants and soothes inflammation.

6. **Witch Hazel:** Acts as a natural toner and astringent.

7. **Clay:** Detoxifies and purifies the skin.

8. **Lemon Juice:** Acts as a natural exfoliant and brightener (use with caution due to photosensitivity).

9. **Jojoba Oil:** Mimics skin's natural sebum and moisturizes.

10. **Shea Butter:** Provides intense moisture and nourishment.

11. **Essential Oils:** Use lavender, tea tree, chamomile, or others for aroma and added benefits.

Caution and Considerations:

- **Allergies:** Be cautious if you have allergies to certain ingredients. Patch-test before applying widely.

- **Skin Sensitivity:** Sensitive skin might react to strong or new ingredients, so choose gentle options.

- **Essential Oils:** Some essential oils can be potent and may require dilution. Research their safe usage.

- **Skin Conditions:** If you have a skin condition like acne or eczema, consult a dermatologist before using DIY products.

- **Photosensitivity:** Some ingredients like lemon juice can make your skin sensitive to sunlight.

DIY beauty and skincare can be a fun and rewarding way to care for your skin and hair using natural ingredients. However, it's important to do your research, be cautious with new ingredients, and consult a professional if you have any concerns about the suitability of a DIY product for your skin type and conditions.

100 tips for effectively using DIY beauty and skincare as a type of home remedy for enhancing your natural beauty:

Getting Started:

1. **Research Ingredients:** Learn about the properties and benefits of various natural ingredients before creating DIY products.

2. **Patch Test:** Always perform a patch test to check for allergic reactions or sensitivities before using a new DIY product on your face or body.

3. **Start Simple:** Begin with basic recipes and gradually experiment with more complex formulations.

4. **Clean Containers:** Ensure the containers and utensils you use are clean to prevent contamination of your DIY products.

5. **Labeling:** Label your DIY products with ingredients and dates to track their freshness.

6. **Fresh Ingredients:** Use fresh and organic ingredients whenever possible for optimal results.

7. **Clean Hands:** Wash your hands thoroughly before preparing and applying DIY products.

8. **Hygiene:** Use clean spatulas or droppers to avoid introducing bacteria into your homemade products.

Facial Care:

9. **Cleansing Oil:** Use oils like jojoba or coconut oil to gently remove makeup and cleanse the face.

10. **Honey Cleanser:** Mix honey with aloe vera or yogurt for a soothing and effective cleanser.

11. **Exfoliating Scrub:** Create a gentle scrub using finely ground oats and honey for mild exfoliation.

12. **Green Tea Toner:** Brew green tea and use it as a refreshing and antioxidant-rich facial toner.

13. **Aloe Vera Gel:** Apply pure aloe vera gel to soothe and hydrate your skin.

14. **Avocado Mask:** Mash avocado and mix with honey for a nourishing face mask.

15. **Turmeric Mask:** Mix turmeric with yogurt and honey for a brightening and clarifying mask.

16. **Cucumber Eye Pads:** Place cucumber slices on your eyes to reduce puffiness and refresh the area.

17. **Rosewater Mist:** Create a DIY rosewater mist to refresh your skin throughout the day.

Lip and Hand Care:

18. **Sugar Lip Scrub:** Make a lip scrub using brown sugar and coconut oil to exfoliate and moisturize lips.

19. **Beeswax Lip Balm:** Mix beeswax, coconut oil, and a few drops of essential oil for homemade lip balm.

20. **Hand Scrub:** Combine sugar and olive oil to create a nourishing hand scrub.

21. **Cuticle Oil:** Use a mixture of jojoba oil and vitamin E oil to soften cuticles.

Hair Care:

22. **Coconut Oil Hair Mask:** Apply coconut oil to your hair for deep conditioning and shine.

23. **Yogurt Hair Mask:** Mix yogurt, honey, and an egg for a protein-rich hair mask.

24. **Apple Cider Vinegar Rinse:** Dilute apple cider vinegar with water and use it as a hair rinse to clarify and add shine.

25. **Aloe Vera Hair Gel:** Apply pure aloe vera gel to style and moisturize your hair.

26. **Herbal Hair Rinse:** Brew herbs like rosemary or chamomile and use the infusion as a hair rinse.

Body Care:

27. **Coffee Body Scrub:** Mix coffee grounds with coconut oil for an invigorating body scrub.

28. **Shea Butter Body Lotion:** Blend shea butter with your favorite essential oils for a moisturizing body lotion.

29. **Milk Bath:** Add powdered milk and a few drops of essential oil to your bath for a nourishing soak.

30. **Soothing Oat Bath:** Place oats in a muslin bag and add it to your bathwater for soothing skin relief.

Sun Protection:

31. **DIY Sunscreen:** Create a natural sunscreen using zinc oxide and coconut oil.

32. **DIY Sunburn Relief:** Apply aloe vera gel mixed with a few drops of lavender essential oil to soothe sunburned skin.

Nail Care:

33. **Cuticle Softener:** Apply a mixture of jojoba oil and vitamin E oil to soften cuticles.

34. **Nail Strengthener:** Soak your nails in a mixture of warm water, lemon juice, and olive oil to strengthen them.

Foot Care:

35. **Foot Scrub:** Exfoliate your feet with a scrub made from sugar and coconut oil.

36. **Peppermint Foot Soak:** Add peppermint essential oil to a foot soak for a refreshing treat.

Special Treatments:

37. **Acne Spot Treatment:** Apply diluted tea tree oil to acne spots for its antibacterial properties.

38. **Under-Eye Treatment:** Place cooled chamomile tea bags on your eyes to reduce puffiness and dark circles.

39. **Teeth Whitening:** Brush your teeth with a mixture of baking soda and water for natural whitening.

Storage and Freshness:

40. **Cool, Dark Place:** Store your DIY products in a cool, dark place to prolong their shelf life.

41. **Small Batches:** Make small batches of DIY products to ensure they stay fresh.

Consultation and Caution:

42. **Allergies:** Be cautious if you have allergies to specific ingredients; avoid them if necessary.

43. **Essential Oil Dilution:** Dilute essential oils properly before using them on your skin.

44. **Consult a Professional:** If you have skin conditions or concerns, consult a dermatologist before using DIY products.

45. **Photosensitivity:** Be aware of photosensitive ingredients like citrus oils that can make your skin sensitive to sunlight.

Body Massage and Relaxation:

46. **Body Oil:** Mix your favorite carrier oils with essential oils for a relaxing and fragrant body massage.

47. **Lavender Pillow Mist:** Create a lavender-infused pillow mist for better sleep and relaxation.

Hair Removal and Shaving:

48. **DIY Sugar Wax:** Make your own sugar wax for natural hair removal.

49. **Shaving Cream:** Mix coconut oil and aloe vera gel for a moisturizing shaving cream.

Personalization:

50. **Customize:** Adjust recipes to suit your skin type, concerns, and fragrance preferences.

51. **Keep Notes:** Keep track of the DIY recipes that work best for you and your skin's needs.

Creative Packaging:

52. **Reuse Containers:** Recycle and repurpose empty containers for storing your DIY products.

53. **Label Creatively:** Decorate your DIY product containers with labels, colors, and designs.

Mindfulness and Self-Care:

54. **Mindful Application:** Apply DIY products mindfully, enjoying the sensory experience.

55. **Self-Care Ritual:** Turn your DIY skincare routine into a self-care ritual to unwind and relax.

Balancing Ingredients:

56. **Balancing Oils:** Choose carrier oils that balance your skin's natural oils rather than making it greasy or dry.

57. **Mix and Match:** Experiment with different combinations of ingredients to find what works best for your skin.

Nature's Remedies:

58. **Herb Infusions:** Create infusions using herbs like calendula, lavender, or chamomile for added benefits.

59. **Flower Petals:** Incorporate dried flower petals like rose or lavender into your DIY products.

Gentle Exfoliation:

60. **Frequency:** Limit exfoliation to a couple of times a week to avoid over-exfoliating your skin.

61. **Gentle Ingredients:** Choose gentle exfoliants like finely ground oats or sugar for facial scrubs.

Anti-Aging Care:

62. **Antioxidant Serums:** Use ingredients like vitamin C and green tea to create antioxidant-rich serums.

Hydration Boost:

63. **Hyaluronic Acid:** Add hyaluronic acid to your DIY products for added hydration.

Healthy Eating:

64. **Hydrate Internally:** Stay hydrated by drinking plenty of water for healthy and glowing skin.

Stress Relief:

65. **Aromatherapy:** Incorporate calming essential oils like lavender into your DIY skincare routine for stress relief.

DIY Hair Styling:

66. **Texturizing Spray:** Create a sea salt spray for natural-looking hair texture and volume.

Holistic Health:

67. **Well-Balanced Diet:** Maintain a balanced diet rich in vitamins, minerals, and antioxidants for overall skin health.

Consistency:

68. **Regular Use:** Use your DIY products consistently to see noticeable results over time.

Mindful Removal:

69. **Gentle Removal:** Be gentle when removing DIY products to avoid irritating your skin.

Expiry Date:

70. **Monitor Freshness:** Keep track of when you made your DIY products and discard them when they expire.

Healthy Lifestyle:

71. **Regular Exercise:** Engage in regular physical activity to promote circulation and healthy skin.

Natural Fragrance:

72. **Essential Oil Perfume:** Create your own natural perfume using essential oils and carrier oils.

Facial Massage:

73. **Lymphatic Drainage:** Incorporate gentle facial massage techniques for lymphatic drainage and relaxation.

Mindful Ingredients:

74. **Check Labels:** Be mindful of the ingredients in store-bought products and choose those with natural ingredients.

Sustainable Choices:

75. **Eco-Friendly Packaging:** Choose reusable and sustainable packaging options for your DIY products.

Simplicity:

76. **Minimal Ingredients:** Embrace simplicity by using products with minimal ingredients for your skincare.

Anti-Inflammatory Care:

77. **Cooling Ingredients:** Use ingredients like cucumber or aloe vera for soothing inflamed skin.

Glowing Skin:

78. **DIY Highlighter:** Mix a small amount of shimmery eyeshadow with aloe vera gel for a natural highlighter.

Natural Fragrance:

79. **DIY Body Spray:** Create a body spray using distilled water and your favorite essential oils.

Mindful Application:

80. **Be Present:** While applying DIY products, focus your attention on the sensation and relaxation it provides.

Self-Love:

81. **Affirmations:** Practice self-love and affirmations while pampering yourself with DIY skincare.

Healthy Fats:

82. **Omega-3 Rich Foods:** Include foods like nuts, seeds, and fatty fish in your diet for healthy skin.

Soothing Remedies:

83. **Aloe Vera Ice Cubes:** Freeze aloe vera gel in ice cube trays and use them to soothe irritated skin.

Beauty Sleep:

84. **Quality Sleep:** Prioritize good quality sleep to allow your skin to rejuvenate naturally.

Calming Rituals:

85. **DIY Bath Bombs:** Create your own bath bombs with calming scents and natural ingredients.

Gentle Cleansing:

86. **No Harsh Scrubbing:** Avoid aggressive scrubbing, especially for facial exfoliation, to prevent irritation.

Healthy Fruits and Veggies:

87. **Vitamin-Rich Diet:** Consume fruits and vegetables rich in vitamins A, C, and E for healthy skin.

Hydrating Masks:

88. **Honey and Yogurt Mask:** Mix honey and yogurt for a hydrating and soothing face mask.

Mindful Showering:

89. **Aromatherapy Shower:** Add a few drops of your favorite essential oil to your shower for an aromatic experience.

Nature's Beauty:

90. **Embrace Natural Beauty:** Use DIY beauty to enhance your natural features rather than covering them up.

Environmentally Friendly:

91. **Zero-Waste Alternatives:** Use DIY products to reduce waste from excessive packaging.

Hair Health:

92. **Scalp Massage:** Incorporate a gentle scalp massage to promote hair health and relaxation.

Refreshing Skin:

93. **DIY Facial Mist:** Create a refreshing mist using rose water or cucumber-infused water.

Meditation:

94. **Mindful Breathing:** Practice deep breathing while applying DIY products for an added sense of calm.

Healthy Mindset:

95. **Positive Thoughts:** Cultivate a positive mindset to radiate beauty from within.

Embrace Imperfections:

96. **Confidence:** Embrace your imperfections and feel confident in your own skin.

Hydrating Drinks:

97. **Herbal Teas:** Enjoy herbal teas like chamomile or hibiscus for internal hydration and glowing skin.

Holistic Well-Being:

98. **Balance:** Remember that beauty is not just skin deep; focus on your holistic well-being.

Joyful Ritual:

99. **Celebrate You:** Make your DIY skincare routine a joyful and self-celebratory ritual.

Gratitude:

100. **Appreciation:** Practice gratitude for your body and skin, nurturing them with love and care.

Remember, DIY beauty and skincare are about nourishing your skin and enhancing your natural beauty. Tailor these tips to your preferences and needs, and enjoy the journey of self-care and self-love.

Teeth and mouth care

Teeth and mouth care as a type of home remedy focuses on maintaining oral hygiene, preventing dental issues, and promoting overall oral health using natural methods and practices. Taking care of your teeth and mouth is crucial not only for a bright smile but also for your overall well-being. Here's a deeper look into teeth and mouth care as a type of home remedy:

Importance of Teeth and Mouth Care:

1. **Oral Health Impact:** Poor oral hygiene can lead to various dental issues, including cavities, gum disease, and bad breath.

2. **Systemic Health:** Oral health is connected to overall health; gum disease has been linked to conditions like diabetes and heart disease.

3. **Confidence:** Good oral hygiene contributes to a confident smile and improved self-esteem.

4. **Preventive Approach:** Home remedies for teeth and mouth care can be a proactive way to prevent dental problems and reduce the need for invasive treatments.

Common Teeth and Mouth Care Practices:

1. **Brushing:** Regularly brushing your teeth using fluoride-free toothpaste and a soft-bristle toothbrush is essential for removing plaque and food particles.

2. **Flossing:** Floss daily to remove debris and plaque from between your teeth where your toothbrush can't reach.

3. **Tongue Cleaning:** Gently scrape your tongue with a tongue scraper or the back of your toothbrush to remove bacteria and improve breath.

4. **Oil Pulling:** Swish coconut or sesame oil in your mouth for 10-20 minutes to remove toxins and promote oral health.

5. **Rinsing:** Use a natural mouthwash or saltwater rinse to reduce bacteria and freshen breath.

6. **Avoid Tobacco:** Avoid smoking or using tobacco products, which can lead to gum disease, bad breath, and oral cancer.

7. **Limit Sugary Foods:** Reduce consumption of sugary foods and drinks that can contribute to cavities.

8. **Hydration:** Drink water to keep your mouth moist and help flush away food particles.

9. **Balanced Diet:** Eat a balanced diet rich in fruits, vegetables, lean proteins, and whole grains for oral and overall health.

10. **Chewing Sugar-Free Gum:** Chewing sugar-free gum can stimulate saliva production and help clean your teeth.

DIY Teeth and Mouth Care Tips:

1. **Natural Toothpaste:** Make your own toothpaste using baking soda, coconut oil, and essential oils like peppermint for freshness.

2. **Activated Charcoal:** Gently brush with activated charcoal to help whiten teeth; use with caution and not excessively.

3. **Herbal Mouthwash:** Create a herbal mouthwash using ingredients like peppermint, chamomile, and sage for a natural rinse.

4. **Teeth-Whitening Paste:** Mix baking soda and lemon juice for a natural teeth-whitening paste; use occasionally and avoid using lemon too often due to its acidity.

5. **Gentle Exfoliation:** Gently rub a strawberry or banana peel on your teeth for mild exfoliation and natural whitening.

6. **Salt and Baking Soda Scrub:** Combine salt and baking soda for a gentle teeth scrub to remove surface stains.

7. **Calcium-Rich Foods:** Include calcium-rich foods like dairy products, leafy greens, and almonds for strong teeth.

8. **Vitamin C Intake:** Consume foods high in vitamin C, like citrus fruits, to promote healthy gums.

9. **Cloves for Toothache:** Apply clove oil or chew on a clove to relieve toothache temporarily.

10. **Cucumber for Fresh Breath:** Chew cucumber slices to freshen your breath naturally.

11. **Drink Herbal Teas:** Certain herbal teas like green tea and chamomile can have anti-inflammatory and antibacterial effects on oral health.

12. **Hydrogen Peroxide Rinse:** Dilute hydrogen peroxide with water and use it as a mouthwash; use caution and avoid swallowing.

13. **Neem and Basil Paste:** Make a paste from neem leaves and basil leaves; both have antibacterial properties for oral health.

14. **Chew on Sesame Seeds:** Chewing sesame seeds can help remove plaque and promote healthy teeth and gums.

15. **Chewing Neem Sticks:** In some cultures, neem sticks are used as a natural toothbrush to clean teeth and gums.

Caution and Considerations:

- **Sensitive Teeth:** Some DIY methods might be abrasive or too harsh for sensitive teeth; use them cautiously or consult a dentist.

- **Acidity:** Citrus fruits and some DIY ingredients can be acidic, potentially causing enamel erosion; use them in moderation.

- **Consult a Dentist:** If you have dental issues, consult a dentist before using DIY methods to ensure they are appropriate for your condition.

- **Allergies:** Be cautious of allergies to certain ingredients; discontinue use if you experience any adverse reactions.

Professional Care:

While home remedies play a role in maintaining oral health, regular dental check-ups and professional cleanings are crucial. Dentists can identify potential issues early, provide expert advice, and perform treatments if needed.

Overall Wellness:

Teeth and mouth care as a home remedy is part of a holistic approach to health. By taking care of your oral health naturally, you contribute to your overall well-being and confidence.

100 tips for effectively using teeth and mouth care as a type of home remedy to promote oral hygiene and overall oral health:

Daily Oral Hygiene:

1. Brush your teeth at least twice a day, using a fluoride-free toothpaste.

2. Use a soft-bristle toothbrush to prevent gum irritation.

3. Brush for at least two minutes, focusing on each tooth surface.

4. Replace your toothbrush every 3-4 months or sooner if bristles are frayed.

5. Floss daily to remove plaque and food particles from between your teeth.

6. Rinse your mouth with water after consuming sugary or acidic foods.

7. Gently brush your tongue to remove bacteria and improve breath.

8. Avoid brushing too aggressively to prevent enamel erosion and gum damage.

9. Consider using an electric toothbrush for efficient cleaning.

10. Teach proper oral hygiene practices to children from a young age.

Natural Mouthwash and Rinses:

11. Use a saltwater rinse to soothe sore gums and reduce bacteria.

12. Create a herbal mouthwash with mint leaves, sage, or chamomile for freshness.

13. Mix equal parts of water and hydrogen peroxide for an antibacterial rinse.

14. Swish coconut oil in your mouth for oil pulling to remove toxins.

15. Add a drop of tea tree oil to water for an antiseptic mouth rinse.

16. Chew on fresh mint leaves or parsley for natural breath freshening.

Teeth-Whitening Techniques:

17. Brush with activated charcoal occasionally for mild teeth whitening.

18. Apply a paste of baking soda and water to gently whiten teeth.

19. Use hydrogen peroxide cautiously as a teeth-whitening agent.

20. Limit consumption of staining foods and drinks like coffee, tea, and red wine.

21. Eat crunchy fruits and vegetables like apples and carrots to naturally clean teeth.

22. Rinse your mouth with water after consuming staining foods.

Natural Toothpaste Alternatives:

23. Make your own fluoride-free toothpaste using baking soda, coconut oil, and essential oils.

24. Use a paste of baking soda and water as a mild tooth-cleaning agent.

25. Mix crushed strawberries with baking soda for a natural teeth-whitening paste.

26. Gently brush your teeth with a banana peel for natural whitening.

27. Opt for toothpaste with natural ingredients like neem and clove oil.

Gum Care:

28. Massage your gums with your fingers to improve circulation.

29. Use a soft toothbrush or a silicone gum stimulator to gently massage your gums.

30. Incorporate vitamin C-rich foods like oranges and strawberries for healthy gums.

Tongue Cleaning:

31. Scrape your tongue using a tongue scraper to remove bacteria and improve breath.

32. Use a spoon as a makeshift tongue scraper if you don't have one.

Dietary Considerations:

33. Consume calcium-rich foods like dairy products, almonds, and leafy greens for strong teeth.

34. Include vitamin D sources like fatty fish and fortified foods for calcium absorption.

35. Eat crunchy fruits and vegetables to stimulate saliva production and clean teeth.

36. Chew sugar-free gum with xylitol to help prevent cavities.

37. Limit sugary and acidic foods and drinks to reduce the risk of cavities.

38. Include probiotic-rich foods like yogurt for oral health benefits.

Natural Remedies for Bad Breath:

39. Chew on fennel seeds, cardamom, or cloves to freshen your breath naturally.

40. Drink green tea, which contains compounds that fight bacteria and improve breath.

41. Eat apples, which can help neutralize bad breath.

42. Stay hydrated by drinking water throughout the day to prevent dry mouth.

Gentle Whitening Scrubs:

43. Mix baking soda and lemon juice to create a gentle teeth-whitening scrub.

44. Combine salt and baking soda for a mild exfoliating teeth scrub.

Nutritional Supplements:

45. Consider taking vitamin C and vitamin D supplements to support oral health.

46. Consult a healthcare professional before taking any supplements.

Cavity Prevention:

47. Use a fluoride-free toothpaste that contains xylitol for cavity prevention.

48. Avoid snacking frequently to reduce the frequency of acid exposure to teeth.

49. Drink water after consuming acidic foods to help neutralize acids.

50. Chewing sugar-free gum after meals can help increase saliva production, which aids in neutralizing acids.

Healthy Lifestyle Habits:

51. Avoid smoking and tobacco products to prevent oral health issues.

52. Reduce alcohol consumption to support healthy gums and oral tissues.

53. Manage stress to prevent teeth grinding and clenching.

54. Protect your teeth from injury during sports with a mouthguard.

Natural Remedies for Toothache:

55. Apply a cold compress to the outside of your cheek for temporary relief.

56. Rinse your mouth with warm salt water to soothe a toothache.

57. Use a clove oil-soaked cotton ball on the affected area for pain relief.

Gum Health Boosters:

58. Chew on neem sticks or twigs, which are traditionally used for oral health in some cultures.

59. Gargle with diluted neem oil for its antibacterial properties.

Oral Health During Pregnancy:

60. Pay extra attention to oral hygiene during pregnancy to prevent pregnancy gingivitis.

61. Consult your dentist about any dental treatments during pregnancy.

DIY Freshening Spray:

62. Create a natural mouth freshening spray using water and a few drops of peppermint essential oil.

63. Carry a small container of cinnamon sticks to chew on for natural breath freshening.

Mindful Chewing:

64. Chew your food thoroughly to aid in digestion and promote saliva production.

Teeth-Strengthening Foods:

65. Incorporate foods rich in phosphorus like eggs, fish, and dairy for strong teeth.

66. Include vitamin K-rich foods like spinach and kale for bone health.

Strengthening Enamel:

67. Consume foods rich in calcium and phosphorus to strengthen tooth enamel.

68. Avoid brushing immediately after consuming acidic foods to prevent enamel erosion.

Natural Antiseptics:

69. Gargle with diluted apple cider vinegar as a natural antiseptic rinse.

Balancing Oral pH:

70. Consume alkaline foods like leafy greens and cucumbers to balance oral pH.

DIY Mouthwash:

71. Mix water, aloe vera gel, and a few drops of peppermint oil for a refreshing mouthwash.

72. Combine water, tea tree oil, and lemon oil for an antibacterial mouthwash.

Soothing Sensitive Gums:

73. Use a toothpaste designed for sensitive teeth if you experience gum sensitivity.

74. Avoid very hot or cold foods if you have sensitive teeth.

Regular Dental Check-ups:

75. Schedule regular dental check-ups and cleanings to detect and prevent issues early.

76. Discuss any concerns or changes with your dentist during your visits.

Natural Remedy for Dry Mouth:

77. Chew on sugar-free gum with xylitol to stimulate saliva production.

78. Sip water throughout the day to keep your mouth moist.

Herbal Teas for Oral Health:

79. Drink herbal teas like chamomile and calendula, known for their anti-inflammatory properties.

80. Enjoy green tea, which contains antioxidants that benefit oral health.

Oil Pulling Routine:

81. Practice oil pulling with coconut oil or sesame oil for oral detoxification.

82. Start with 5 minutes of oil pulling and gradually increase the duration.

Enamel-Friendly Snacks:

83. Snack on cheese, which can help neutralize acids and promote saliva production.

84. Eat nuts, which provide healthy fats and support oral health.

Mindful Dental Care:

85. Practice mindfulness while brushing and flossing, focusing on each tooth.

Natural Remedy for Cold Sores:

86. Apply aloe vera gel to cold sores for soothing relief.

87. Use a drop of tea tree oil on a cotton swab for antiseptic properties.

Fruits for Oral Health:

88. Consume citrus fruits for vitamin C, which supports gum health.

89. Eat strawberries, which contain malic acid to naturally whiten teeth.

DIY Herbal Tooth Powder:

90. Create a tooth powder using ground dried herbs like sage and peppermint.

91. Gently brush your teeth with the herbal tooth powder for freshness.

Balancing Bacteria:

92. Consume probiotic-rich foods like yogurt to support a healthy oral microbiome.

Gum Health Tea:

93. Brew a tea with cinnamon, cloves, and sage for gum health benefits.

Avoiding Teeth-Staining Foods:

94. Limit consumption of dark-colored foods like berries that can stain teeth.

95. Use a straw when drinking staining beverages to minimize contact with teeth.

Staying Hydrated:

96. Drink water throughout the day to prevent dry mouth and support oral health.

Oral Hygiene for Kids:

97. Teach children proper brushing and flossing techniques from an early age.

98. Make dental hygiene fun for kids with themed toothbrushes and playful routines.

Regular Mouth Muscle Exercises:

99. Practice tongue exercises to improve tongue posture and oral muscle strength.

Positive Mindset for Oral Health:

100. Cultivate a positive attitude towards oral health to motivate consistent care.

Remember that maintaining oral health is an ongoing process. Incorporate these tips into your daily routine to achieve optimal oral hygiene and overall oral health. Regular dental visits are also essential for professional assessment and treatments when necessary.

Naturopathic remedies

Naturopathic remedies, as a type of home remedy, are rooted in the principles of naturopathic medicine, which emphasizes the body's inherent ability to heal itself through natural methods and treatments. Naturopathic remedies encompass a wide range of practices that focus on holistic health, addressing the physical, mental, and emotional aspects of an individual's well-being. Here's a deeper look into naturopathic remedies as a type of home remedy:

Principles of Naturopathic Medicine:

1. **Healing Power of Nature:** Naturopathic remedies believe in the body's natural healing ability and aim to support and enhance it.

2. **Identify and Treat the Cause:** Naturopaths seek to identify and address the root causes of health issues rather than merely treating symptoms.

3. **Do No Harm:** Naturopathic remedies prioritize using methods that minimize harm and avoid suppressing the body's natural processes.

4. **Treat the Whole Person:** Naturopathic medicine recognizes the interconnectedness of physical, mental, emotional, and spiritual health.

5. **Doctor as Teacher:** Naturopaths educate and empower individuals to take charge of their health through informed decisions.

6. **Prevention:** Prevention is key in naturopathic medicine, focusing on maintaining optimal health and preventing disease.

7. **Individualized Care:** Naturopathic remedies are tailored to each person's unique needs and constitution.

Types of Naturopathic Remedies:

1. **Diet and Nutrition:** Nutrition is central to naturopathic remedies. Practitioners emphasize whole foods, balanced diets, and addressing deficiencies.

2. **Herbal Medicine:** Using plants and botanicals for their healing properties is a cornerstone of naturopathic remedies.

3. **Supplements:** Nutritional supplements may be recommended to address specific deficiencies or support overall health.

4. **Homeopathy:** This practice involves using highly diluted substances to stimulate the body's healing response.

5. **Hydrotherapy:** Hydrotherapy uses water in various forms (hot and cold compresses, baths) to support healing and detoxification.

6. **Physical Manipulation:** Techniques like chiropractic adjustments and osteopathic manipulation are used to improve musculoskeletal health.

7. **Mind-Body Techniques:** Mindfulness, meditation, and relaxation techniques are used to promote emotional and mental well-being.

8. **Lifestyle Counseling:** Naturopaths offer guidance on adopting healthy lifestyle practices, stress management, and sleep hygiene.

9. **Exercise:** Physical activity is promoted for its benefits to cardiovascular health, mood, and overall well-being.

10. **Detoxification:** Methods to support the body's detoxification processes are utilized, such as saunas and herbal cleanses.

Common Naturopathic Remedies:

1. **Echinacea:** Used to support the immune system during colds and infections.

2. **Ginger:** Known for its anti-inflammatory and digestive benefits.

3. **Turmeric:** Used as an anti-inflammatory and antioxidant.

4. **Chamomile:** Promotes relaxation and is often used for digestive issues.

5. **Peppermint:** Supports digestion and may help with headaches.

6. **Lavender:** Used for its calming and stress-relieving properties.

7. **Probiotics:** Supports gut health and the immune system.

8. **Epsom Salt Baths:** Used for relaxation and to promote detoxification.

9. **Castor Oil Packs:** Applied topically for detoxification and pain relief.

10. **Arnica:** Used topically for bruising and muscle soreness.

11. **Feverfew:** Often used for migraines and headaches.

12. **Valerian:** Used for its calming and sleep-promoting effects.

13. **Bach Flower Remedies:** These flower essences are used to address emotional imbalances.

Applying Naturopathic Remedies at Home:

1. **Holistic Nutrition:** Focus on a balanced diet rich in whole foods, vegetables, and lean proteins.

2. **Herbal Teas:** Incorporate herbal teas like chamomile, peppermint, or ginger for specific benefits.

3. **Mindful Eating:** Practice mindful eating, paying attention to hunger and satiety cues.

4. **Essential Oils:** Use essential oils like lavender or eucalyptus for aromatherapy or topical applications.

5. **Hydrotherapy:** Take contrast showers or warm baths with Epsom salts for relaxation.

6. **Yoga and Meditation:** Incorporate yoga and meditation for stress reduction and improved mental well-being.

7. **Lifestyle Adjustments:** Focus on stress reduction, quality sleep, and regular physical activity.

8. **Mind-Body Connection:** Cultivate practices that promote a positive mind-body connection.

Considerations and Precautions:

- **Consult a Professional:** Before starting any naturopathic remedy, consult a qualified naturopathic doctor or healthcare provider, especially if you have underlying health conditions or are taking medications.

- **Individualized Approach:** Naturopathic remedies are often tailored to an individual's specific needs; what works for one person might not work for another.

- **Interaction with Conventional Treatments:** Inform your healthcare provider about any naturopathic remedies you're using to ensure they don't interact negatively with prescribed medications.

- **Allergies and Sensitivities:** Be aware of potential allergies or sensitivities to herbs, essential oils, or other natural substances.

Overall Philosophy:

Naturopathic remedies encourage a balanced approach to health and healing. While these remedies can be effective, they are best used in conjunction with conventional medical care when necessary. Practicing naturopathic remedies at home can be a proactive way to support your health and well-being in a holistic manner.

100 tips for effectively using naturopathic remedies as a type of home remedy to promote holistic health and well-being:

Diet and Nutrition:

1. Consume a variety of whole foods, including fruits, vegetables, whole grains, and lean proteins.

2. Choose organic produce when possible to reduce exposure to pesticides.

3. Incorporate fermented foods like yogurt and sauerkraut to support gut health.

4. Reduce processed foods and sugar intake for overall well-being.

5. Stay hydrated by drinking plenty of water throughout the day.

6. Use herbs and spices like turmeric, garlic, and ginger for added flavor and health benefits.

7. Opt for healthy fats from sources like avocados, nuts, and olive oil.

Herbal Medicine:

8. Research and consult a professional before using herbs for specific health concerns.

9. Enjoy herbal teas like chamomile, peppermint, and nettle for various benefits.

10. Create herbal tinctures using alcohol or glycerin to extract medicinal properties.

11. Use calendula salve for skin irritations and minor wounds.

12. Incorporate adaptogenic herbs like ashwagandha and rhodiola for stress support.

Supplements:

13. Consult a healthcare provider before taking any supplements to address deficiencies.

14. Consider vitamin D supplementation, especially in the winter months.

15. Choose high-quality supplements from reputable brands for better absorption.

Homeopathy:

16. Consult a trained homeopath to identify appropriate remedies for specific symptoms.

17. Use Arnica montana for bruises and minor injuries.

18. Try Chamomilla for teething discomfort in babies.

19. Use Nux vomica for digestive issues related to overindulgence.

Hydrotherapy:

20. Take warm baths with Epsom salts to relax muscles and promote detoxification.

21. Alternate between warm and cold compresses to boost circulation and immunity.

22. Use warm water foot baths with ginger for cold relief.

Physical Manipulation:

23. Consider chiropractic adjustments for musculoskeletal issues and spinal health.

24. Explore osteopathic manipulation for pain relief and improved mobility.

Mind-Body Techniques:

25. Practice deep breathing exercises for stress reduction and relaxation.

26. Engage in daily meditation to improve focus and mental clarity.

27. Try progressive muscle relaxation for tension release.

Lifestyle Counseling:

28. Establish a regular sleep routine to support restful sleep.

29. Manage stress through mindfulness, yoga, or Tai Chi.

30. Spend time in nature for improved mood and well-being.

Exercise:

31. Engage in regular physical activity, such as walking, yoga, or swimming.

32. Incorporate stretching to improve flexibility and prevent muscle tension.

Detoxification:

33. Consume fiber-rich foods to support natural detoxification processes.

34. Stay hydrated with water and herbal teas to flush toxins from the body.

Holistic Mindset:

35. Embrace a holistic view of health, considering physical, mental, and emotional aspects.

36. Cultivate a positive mindset through affirmations and self-care practices.

Personalized Care:

37. Tailor naturopathic remedies to your individual needs and preferences.

38. Seek guidance from a qualified naturopathic doctor for a personalized approach.

Positive Attitude:

39. Maintain a positive attitude toward healing and trust in your body's abilities.

40. Practice gratitude to enhance your overall well-being.

Mindful Eating:

41. Eat mindfully, paying attention to hunger and fullness cues.

42. Avoid distractions like screens while eating to fully savor your meals.

Herbal Baths:

43. Add soothing herbs like lavender or chamomile to your bathwater for relaxation.

44. Use oatmeal baths to soothe irritated skin.

Nourishing Teas:

45. Brew teas with elderberry, echinacea, and ginger for immune support.

46. Enjoy calming teas like passionflower and valerian for relaxation.

Nurturing Sleep:

47. Create a calming bedtime routine to promote restful sleep.

48. Use lavender essential oil in a diffuser to enhance relaxation before sleep.

Holistic Stress Relief:

49. Practice yoga or deep breathing techniques to manage stress and anxiety.

50. Connect with nature through outdoor walks or gardening for stress reduction.

Natural Topical Treatments:

51. Apply aloe vera gel for skin irritations and sunburn relief.

52. Use tea tree oil diluted in carrier oil for blemishes and minor skin infections.

Mindful Meditation:

53. Start your day with a short meditation to set a positive tone.

54. Practice mindfulness meditation during stressful moments.

Nutrient-Rich Foods:

55. Include dark leafy greens like spinach and kale for their nutrient density.

56. Eat colorful fruits and vegetables for a wide range of vitamins and minerals.

Proper Hydration:

57. Drink herbal teas and infused water for added hydration and flavor.

58. Consume electrolyte-rich foods like coconut water for hydration.

Outdoor Time:

59. Spend time in natural sunlight to support vitamin D production and mood.

60. Practice grounding by walking barefoot on grass or soil.

Holistic Dental Care:

61. Use natural toothpaste without fluoride or artificial additives.

62. Try oil pulling with coconut oil for oral health and detoxification.

Healthy Oils:

63. Cook with coconut oil or olive oil for their health benefits.

64. Use flaxseed oil for its omega-3 fatty acids.

Energetic Healing:

65. Explore energy healing practices like Reiki or acupuncture for balance.

66. Practice qigong or tai chi for cultivating energy flow.

Plant-Based Eating:

67. Consider adopting a plant-based diet for its health and environmental benefits.

68. Incorporate plant-based proteins like beans, lentils, and quinoa.

Holistic Digestive Health:

69. Consume fiber-rich foods like whole grains and legumes for gut health.

70. Include fermented foods like kimchi and kefir for a healthy gut microbiome.

Natural Pain Relief:

71. Apply arnica gel topically for muscle soreness and bruises.

72. Use essential oils like peppermint or lavender for tension headaches.

Holistic Skincare:

73. Create a DIY face mask with natural ingredients like honey and yogurt.

74. Use rosehip oil for its skin-nourishing properties.

Emotional Wellness:

75. Practice journaling as a tool for self-expression and emotional processing.

76. Engage in creative activities like painting or playing a musical instrument.

Mindful Movement:

77. Incorporate mindful movement practices like tai chi or qigong.

78. Try forest bathing—a mindful walk in nature—for relaxation.

Holistic Immune Support:

79. Include immune-boosting foods like citrus fruits and garlic in your diet.

80. Practice gentle movement or yoga to support lymphatic circulation.

Holistic Respiratory Health:

81. Use eucalyptus essential oil in a diffuser to promote clear breathing.

82. Stay hydrated and consume warm herbal teas for respiratory comfort.

Holistic Skin Health:

83. Stay hydrated to promote healthy skin from the inside out.

84. Use natural exfoliants like oatmeal or sugar for gentle skin exfoliation.

Holistic Hormone Balance:

85. Incorporate foods rich in omega-3 fatty acids for hormonal support.

86. Manage stress through meditation or gentle exercise to support hormonal balance.

Holistic Cardiovascular Health:

87. Eat heart-healthy foods like nuts, seeds, and fatty fish.

88. Engage in regular cardiovascular exercise for heart health.

Holistic Mental Clarity:

89. Consume omega-3-rich foods like walnuts and chia seeds for brain health.

90. Practice mindfulness meditation to improve focus and mental clarity.

Holistic Joint Health:

91. Include anti-inflammatory foods like turmeric and berries in your diet.

92. Try gentle yoga or swimming to support joint flexibility.

Holistic Energy Boost:

93. Consume complex carbohydrates for sustained energy throughout the day.

94. Use invigorating essential oils like citrus or peppermint for energy.

Holistic Digestive Comfort:

95. Enjoy herbal teas like peppermint or ginger for soothing digestive discomfort.

96. Practice deep breathing exercises to ease digestive tension.

Holistic Stress Relief:

97. Listen to soothing music or nature sounds to unwind and reduce stress.

98. Create a calming environment with dim lighting and comfortable surroundings.

Holistic Sleep Support:

99. Establish a bedtime routine with relaxation techniques to promote better sleep.

100. Use calming herbal teas like chamomile or valerian before bed to enhance sleep quality.

Remember, naturopathic remedies work best as part of a comprehensive approach to health. Consulting a qualified healthcare provider before making significant changes to your health regimen is important, especially if you have underlying health conditions or are taking medications.

Folk remedies

Folk remedies, also known as traditional or folkloric remedies, are age-old healing practices and treatments that have been passed down through generations within specific cultures or communities. These remedies are often based on local knowledge, experience, and observations of the natural world. Folk remedies are deeply rooted in cultural traditions and reflect the wisdom and resourcefulness of past generations. Here's a closer look at folk remedies as a type of home remedy:

Cultural and Regional Diversity:

1. **Variety of Approaches:** Folk remedies vary widely based on cultural, regional, and ethnic backgrounds. Different cultures have their own unique remedies for common ailments.

2. **Plant-Based Remedies:** Many folk remedies utilize plants and herbs that are native to the region, often foraged from the local environment.

3. **Tradition and Ritual:** Folk remedies often come with specific rituals, chants, or practices that are believed to enhance their effectiveness.

4. **Oral Tradition:** These remedies are typically passed down orally from one generation to another, fostering a sense of community and connection.

5. **Community Healing:** Folk remedies often promote a communal approach to healing, where knowledge is shared within the community.

Common Folk Remedies:

6. **Hot Water and Lemon:** Consuming warm water with lemon is a common remedy for promoting digestion and detoxification.

7. **Honey and Lemon for Sore Throat:** Mixing honey and lemon in warm water is used to soothe a sore throat.

8. **Onion Poultice:** Applying a poultice made from grated onions on the chest is believed to help with respiratory congestion.

9. **Garlic for Immunity:** Garlic is often consumed to boost immunity and fight infections.

10. **Saltwater Gargle:** Gargling with warm saltwater is used to relieve a sore throat.

11. **Mustard Plaster:** Applying a mustard plaster to the chest is believed to help with congestion and respiratory issues.

12. **Rice Water for Diarrhea:** Drinking rice water is a traditional remedy to soothe diarrhea.

13. **Ginger for Nausea:** Consuming ginger tea or ginger-infused water is used to alleviate nausea.

14. **Turmeric for Inflammation:** Turmeric is often used as an anti-inflammatory agent and is believed to have healing properties.

15. **Epsom Salt Bath:** Taking a bath with Epsom salts is a popular remedy for relaxation and muscle soreness.

Natural Ingredients:

16. **Kitchen Ingredients:** Folk remedies often utilize common kitchen ingredients like honey, vinegar, garlic, and spices.

17. **Herbs and Plants:** Many folk remedies rely on the healing properties of locally available herbs and plants.

18. **Bone Broth:** Homemade bone broth is believed to have restorative properties for overall health.

19. **Mud and Clay:** Topical application of mud or clay is used for skin issues and inflammation.

20. **Comfrey:** Comfrey leaves are applied topically to promote wound healing.

21. **Plantain Leaf:** Plantain leaves are used as a natural remedy for insect bites and skin irritations.

Regional Wisdom:

22. **Aloe Vera for Burns:** Aloe vera gel is commonly applied to soothe burns and minor skin irritations.

23. **Chamomile Tea:** Drinking chamomile tea is believed to aid digestion and promote relaxation.

24. **Nettle Tea:** Nettle tea is often used to relieve allergies and support kidney function.

25. **Fennel Seeds for Digestion:** Chewing fennel seeds is believed to aid digestion and freshen breath.

26. **Bitter Herbs for Digestion:** Consuming bitter herbs like dandelion or gentian root is thought to stimulate digestion.

27. **Horse Chestnut for Varicose Veins:** Horse chestnut extract is used as a natural remedy for varicose veins.

Traditional Practices:

28. **Cupping Therapy:** Cupping involves creating suction on the skin to stimulate blood flow and promote healing.

29. **Acupressure:** Applying pressure to specific points on the body to alleviate pain and promote healing.

30. **Foot Reflexology:** Stimulating specific areas of the feet is believed to impact various organs and systems.

31. **Hot and Cold Therapy:** Alternating between hot and cold treatments is used to reduce inflammation and promote circulation.

Historical Wisdom:

32. **Cod Liver Oil:** Cod liver oil was traditionally consumed for its vitamins A and D content.

33. **Cranberry Juice for UTIs:** Drinking cranberry juice is believed to help prevent urinary tract infections.

34. **Honey and Cinnamon:** A mixture of honey and cinnamon is used in various cultures for different health benefits.

35. **Essential Oils:** Aromatherapy using essential oils is a traditional practice for emotional and physical well-being.

36. **Cultural Context:** Folk remedies often come from specific cultural contexts, and their efficacy may vary based on individual beliefs.

37. **Research and Modern Science:** Some folk remedies align with modern scientific understanding, while others may lack scientific evidence.

38. **Individual Reactions:** Just like with any remedy, individual reactions can vary, and what works for one person might not work for another.

39. **Consulting Professionals:** It's important to consult with healthcare professionals before trying new remedies, especially for serious health concerns.

40. **Balancing Tradition and Modern Medicine:** Folk remedies can complement modern medical treatments, but it's crucial to strike a balance and make informed decisions.

Folk remedies hold a rich cultural heritage and offer insights into the ways different communities have approached health and well-being over the years. While some remedies might be based on tradition and anecdotal evidence, others align with modern scientific understanding. Integrating folk remedies with evidence-based medical practices can provide a holistic approach to health and wellness.

100 tips for effectively using folk remedies as a type of home remedy to promote health and well-being. Remember that while many of these remedies have been used for generations, it's important to consult with a healthcare professional before trying new treatments, especially for serious health concerns.

General Folk Remedies:

1. Research and understand the specific folk remedy before trying it.

2. Respect cultural practices and traditions associated with the remedy.

3. Share your folk remedies and stories with your family to keep the tradition alive.

4. Approach folk remedies with an open mind and willingness to learn from different cultures.

5. Be patient and consistent with folk remedies, as results might take time.

Herbal Remedies:

6. Infuse herbs in warm water to create herbal teas for various health benefits.

7. Grow your own medicinal herbs at home for easy access.

8. Learn about the properties of different herbs and their traditional uses.

9. Use herbal poultices or compresses for localized healing.

10. Incorporate dried herbs into your cooking for added flavor and health benefits.

Kitchen Ingredients:

11. Use honey to soothe sore throats or as an antibacterial agent for minor cuts.

12. Consume a teaspoon of apple cider vinegar for digestive support.

13. Apply coconut oil to dry skin or hair for moisturizing benefits.

14. Create a soothing face mask using yogurt and turmeric for skin radiance.

15. Use baking soda as a gentle exfoliant for skin and teeth.

Natural Substances:

16. Apply aloe vera gel to sunburned skin for relief.

17. Use olive oil to moisturize dry skin or as a base for herbal infusions.

18. Apply cucumber slices to tired eyes to reduce puffiness.

19. Soak in a bath with Epsom salts to ease muscle soreness.

Kitchen Remedies:

20. Drink warm milk with honey to aid sleep.

21. Consume a spoonful of honey for a natural energy boost.

22. Eat a banana for a quick source of potassium and energy.

23. Use a slice of raw onion to ease insect stings and bites.

24. Mix salt and warm water for a simple gargle to soothe a sore throat.

Spices and Herbs:

25. Chew on fennel seeds after meals to aid digestion.

26. Sprinkle cinnamon on oatmeal or toast for its warming properties.

27. Brew ginger tea to alleviate nausea and support digestion.

28. Use garlic as a natural antimicrobial and immune booster.

29. Mix turmeric with warm milk for its anti-inflammatory benefits.

Cold and Flu Remedies:

30. Inhale steam with eucalyptus oil to relieve congestion.

31. Make a hot ginger and honey drink to soothe a sore throat.

32. Sip on warm herbal teas like chamomile or peppermint for comfort.

33. Place a slice of onion by your bedside to alleviate cold symptoms.

Digestive Health:

34. Drink peppermint tea to ease indigestion and bloating.

35. Consume yogurt for its probiotic benefits to support gut health.

36. Chew on caraway seeds to relieve gas and bloating.

37. Sip warm water with lemon in the morning to aid digestion.

Skin and Hair Care:

38. Use oatmeal for a soothing bath to calm irritated skin.

39. Apply a paste of turmeric and honey for its antibacterial properties.

40. Use tea tree oil diluted in water as a natural toner for acne-prone skin.

41. Massage coconut oil into your scalp for nourishment and hydration.

Stress and Relaxation:

42. Practice deep breathing exercises to reduce stress and anxiety.

43. Brew chamomile tea before bedtime to promote relaxation.

44. Use lavender essential oil in a diffuser for a calming atmosphere.

45. Try meditation or mindfulness practices for stress relief.

Energy and Vitality:

46. Snack on nuts and dried fruits for a quick energy boost.

47. Drink green tea for its natural caffeine content and antioxidants.

48. Enjoy a balanced breakfast with protein and complex carbohydrates for sustained energy.

Immune Support:

49. Consume vitamin C-rich foods like citrus fruits for immune health.

50. Make a garlic and honey syrup for immune-boosting benefits.

51. Use echinacea tea during cold and flu seasons for immune support.

Joint and Muscle Care:

52. Apply a mixture of turmeric and warm milk to ease joint discomfort.

53. Use ginger oil in a massage blend for muscle soreness.

54. Create a poultice with crushed comfrey leaves for muscle relief.

Hair Health:

55. Rinse hair with diluted apple cider vinegar for shine and scalp health.

56. Use aloe vera gel on the scalp to soothe irritation and dandruff.

57. Apply henna for a natural hair dye and conditioning treatment.

Sleep Support:

58. Create a bedtime routine to signal your body for sleep.

59. Drink valerian root tea for its calming and sleep-inducing properties.

60. Use lavender sachets under your pillow for relaxation.

Hydration and Detox:

61. Drink warm lemon water in the morning to support detoxification.

62. Stay hydrated by drinking water throughout the day.

63. Enjoy herbal teas with dandelion or nettle for gentle detox support.

Mindfulness and Well-Being:

64. Practice grounding by walking barefoot on natural surfaces.

65. Spend time in nature to recharge and improve mental well-being.

66. Try forest bathing—a mindful walk in the woods—for relaxation.

Oral Health:

67. Use oil pulling with coconut or sesame oil for oral health.

68. Chew on parsley leaves to naturally freshen your breath.

69. Rinse your mouth with warm saltwater to soothe oral irritations.

Fertility and Women's Health:

70. Drink raspberry leaf tea to support women's reproductive health.

71. Apply castor oil packs to the abdomen to promote circulation and relaxation.

72. Consume iron-rich foods like spinach to support menstrual health.

Children's Health:

73. Use a warm compress with chamomile tea for colicky infants.

74. Offer honey for its soothing properties during coughs in children over one year old.

75. Apply diluted lavender oil to a child's pillow for a calming sleep environment.

Eye Health:

76. Apply cooled chamomile tea bags to soothe tired eyes.

77. Use cucumber slices to reduce puffiness and refresh the eyes.

Natural Immunity Boosters:

78. Consume elderberry syrup or tea during cold and flu seasons.

79. Eat foods rich in zinc, like pumpkin seeds, for immune support.

Traditional Healing Practices:

80. Explore traditional practices like acupuncture or cupping for holistic healing.

81. Incorporate acupressure or reflexology techniques for relaxation and well-being.

Balancing Hot and Cold:

82. Use hot water bottles or warm compresses for pain relief.

83. Apply cold packs to reduce inflammation and alleviate swelling.

Mindful Eating:

84. Pay attention to the textures and flavors of your food to enhance digestion.

85. Chew your food thoroughly to support proper digestion and absorption.

Natural Cleaning Solutions:

86. Use vinegar and water as a natural cleaning solution for surfaces.

87. Sprinkle baking soda on carpets before vacuuming for odor removal.

Heritage and Cultural Connection:

88. Learn about your own cultural heritage's folk remedies and their benefits.

89. Share folk remedies and stories with friends and family to maintain cultural connections.

Respectful Approach:

90. Approach folk remedies with an attitude of respect and curiosity.

91. Understand that what works for one person might not work for another due to individual differences.

Mind-Body Practices:

92. Combine folk remedies with mindfulness practices for a holistic approach to well-being.

93. Practice yoga or tai chi to enhance the mind-body connection.

Healthy Aging:

94. Consume foods rich in antioxidants to support healthy aging.

95. Stay physically active and engage in mental exercises to maintain cognitive health.

Balanced Diet:

96. Consume a variety of nutrient-rich foods to support overall health.

97. Incorporate fermented foods like kimchi for gut health and digestion.

Connecting with Nature:

98. Use herbal remedies as a way to connect with the natural world.

99. Practice forest therapy or earthing to enhance your connection with nature.

Consultation and Moderation:

100. Consult with healthcare professionals before trying new folk remedies, especially for serious health concerns.

Use folk remedies in moderation and balance them with evidence-based medical practices.

Folk remedies can be a wonderful way to connect with ancestral wisdom and incorporate traditional practices into your modern lifestyle. While these remedies have been used for generations, it's important to approach them with an open mind, gather knowledge from reliable sources, and consult with healthcare professionals when needed.